SPA JOURNEYS

for Body Mind and Soul

Photographs by LINDA TROELLER Text by ANNETTE FOGLINO

pH powerHouse Books New York, NY

CONTENTS

SPAS, UNITED STATES

PRICE GUIDELINES

$	$100–200	Price is based on approximate cost of room per day, per person, double occupancy, plus three meals and one spa treatment during high season.
$$	$200–300	
$$$	$300–400	
$$$$	$400–500	
$$$$$	$500+	

SPAS, INTERNATIONAL

ROOM CATEGORY DESCRIPTIONS

Basic, clean & pleasant
A quite acceptable, but unspectacular, hotel room.
Elegantly appointed
A fine room with decorative touches such as
antiques or fresh flowers.
Sumptuous and luxurious
A beautiful room with extra special touches, such as
opulent down comforters or gorgeous marble tubs.

The prices listed in this book were confirmed at
press time but under no circumstances are they
guaranteed. We recommend contacting the
establishments for current information.

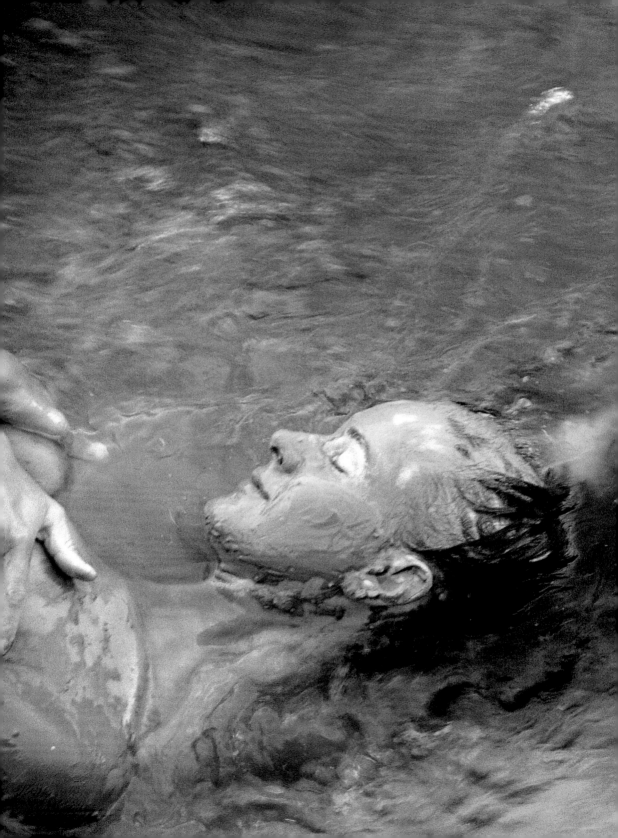

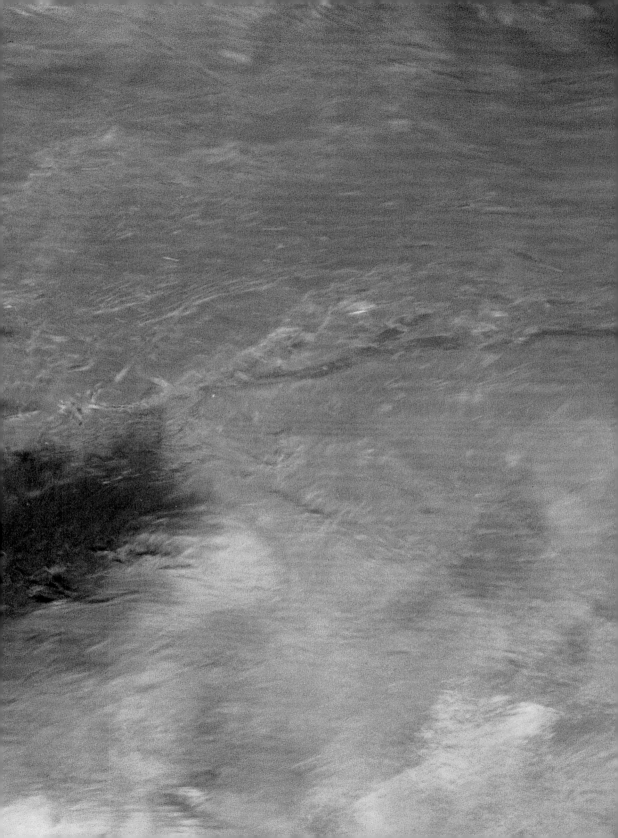

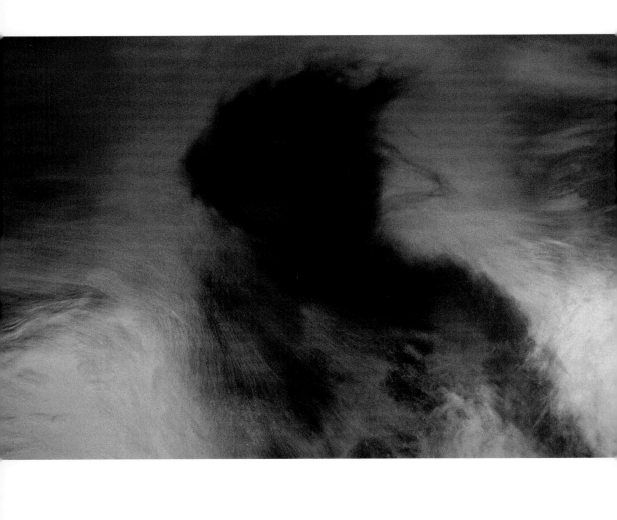

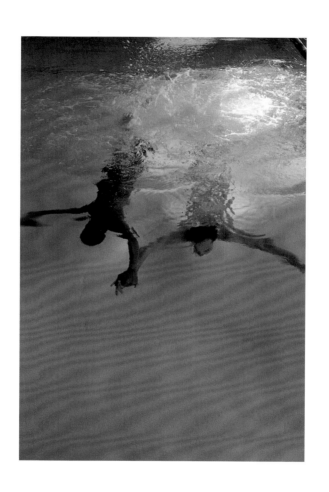

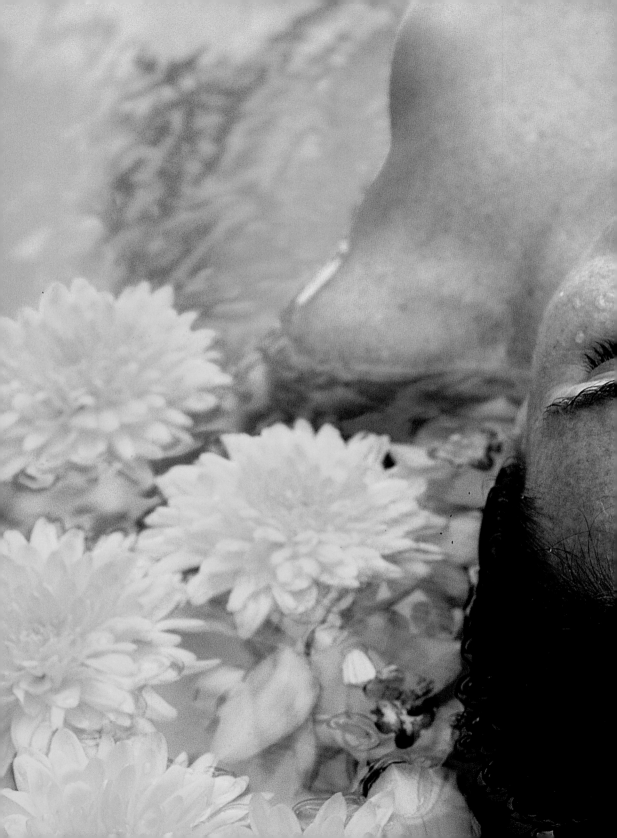

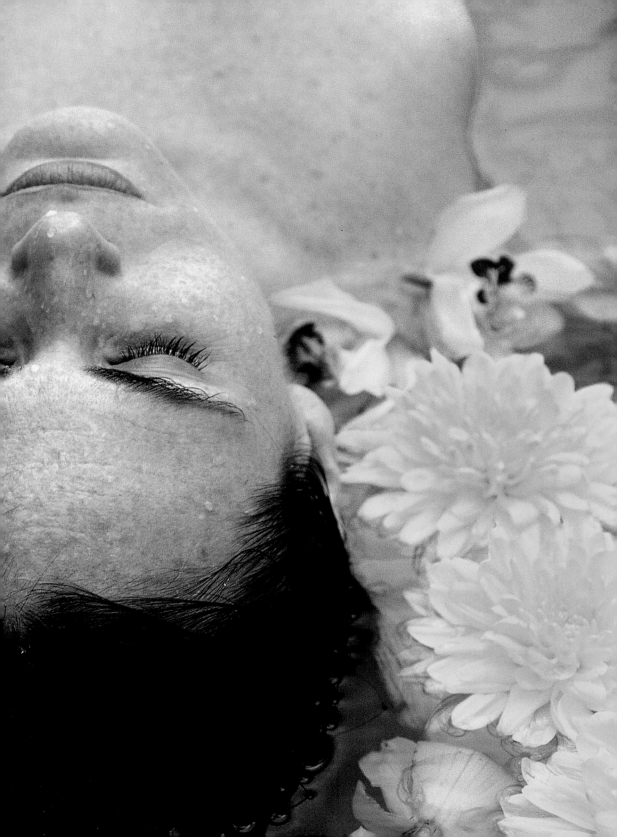

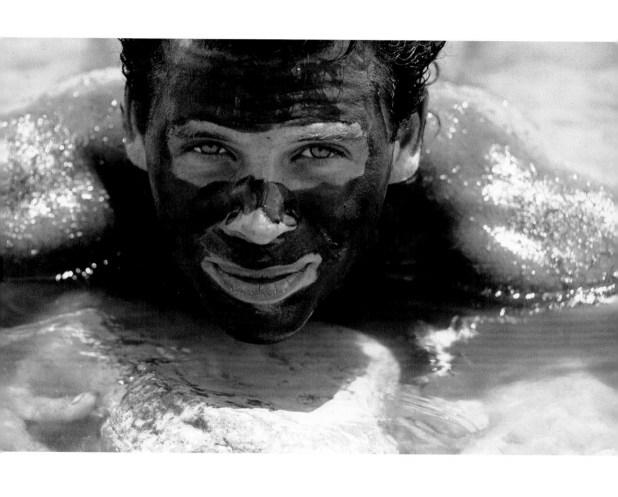

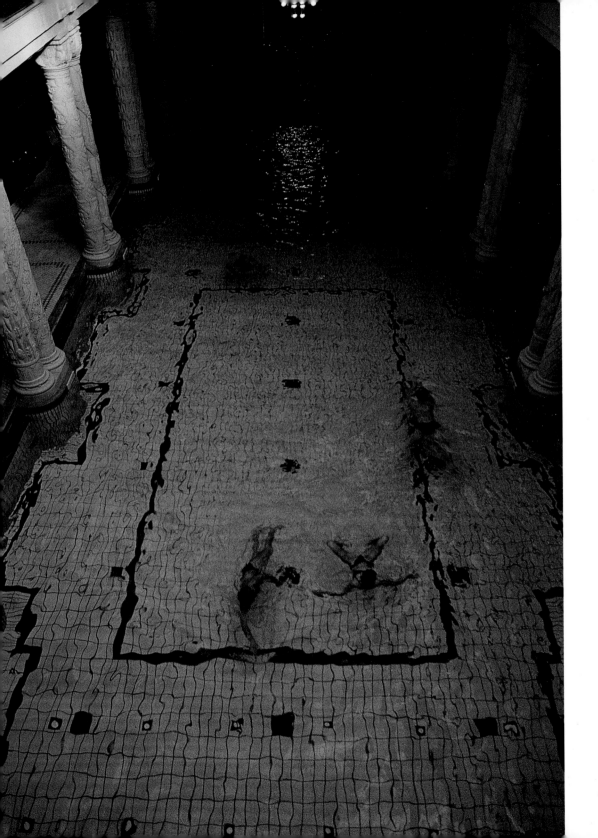

INTRODUCTION

In a Native American parable, the Creator gathers all the animals and says: "I want to hide something from humans until they are ready for it—the realization that they create their own reality."

> *"Give it to me. I'll fly it to the moon," says the eagle.*
>
> *"No, one day soon they will go there and find it."*
>
> *"How about at the bottom of the ocean?" asks the salmon.*
>
> *"No, they will find it there too."*
>
> *"I will bury it in the great plains," says the buffalo.*
>
> *"They will soon dig and find it there."*
>
> *"Put it inside them," says wise grandmother mole.*
>
> *"Done," says the Creator. "It is the last place they will look."*

One of the great wonders of travel is that a journey far from home can actually take us deep inside ourselves. When we surround ourselves with new locations, the dusty tangles of everyday worries and responsibilities drop away, and we see our lives in a new light. With this release, a vacation becomes much more than just "time off." After all, the word *vacation* comes from the Latin word *vacare*, which means "to be empty or free." A spa journey is the quickest, most effective—and if you choose, most luxurious—route to this very special kind of freedom. It not only offers an opportunity to "empty" yourself, but to fill up with more positive ways of being.

Linda Troeller, the photographer for this book, first visited a spa twenty years ago. "I was going through this awful breakup and I went to Mexico to do black-and-white photography—I was a student of Ansel Adams and that was what all the art photographers were doing at the time," she says. Once there, Linda's mind was still centered on her relationship, trying to fathom why it wasn't working. "I met the great surrealist painter Leonora Carrington and she said to me, 'You can't be sad in Mexico. You should try some magic mushrooms or visit some hot springs.'" Linda decided to pass on the mushrooms, but she did go to a spa in Ixtapan, Mexico. There, a local Indian healer led her to a treatment room in which little jars of mud lined the walls. The healer told her to cover her body with the mud. "It will draw all your sins from you," she said. "And the water from the hot springs will wash them all away."

Linda bathed in the springs every day for a week, and copied the local Indians, taking the water in her cupped hands and pouring it over her heart. As the week passed, she had a few cries and plenty of rest. Her energy and optimism began to return and, with them, a renewed appetite for life. "I had been at a crossroads in my art, too," she says. "But I saw new possibilities. I decided to learn more about hot springs and healing sites and capture them on film. When I got home, I was also able to face the end of my relationship with a little more peace. I was ready to let it go." Like millions before her, Linda had discovered the rejuvenating power of spa life.

Many Americans still think of spas as places to go to have their toenails buffed, or their eyelids draped with cucumber slices, or to starve themselves into twigginess on a diet of steamed lettuce leaves. Personally, I've never encountered a facialist holding anything resembling a cucumber (though I have seen the vegetable used in foot baths), and most spa food is anything but Spartan nowadays. You can begin the day with stuffed French toast and end it with a chocolate napoleon dessert. A spa journey has become about much more than shedding fat and getting a good massage. In this day and age, everyone knows that dieting is not the answer to a weight problem. Losing weight and keeping it off requires a change in lifestyle.

In the last two decades, millions of people have become interested in self-improvement and transformation, and have recognized that spas are among the best places to make progress in these pursuits. Spas have become like academies, where visitors train themselves in the art of living. At many, wherever you turn, there is a yoga or meditation class, a seminar on the latest relaxation techniques, or a lecture from a renowned mind-body expert. You can even star in your own private Oprah or Dr. Phil show and hash out problems that have plagued you for years.

When I began writing about spas almost ten years ago, I had never had a massage or a facial. At first I found these treatments a little boring, and I hated the phrases "let go" and "take a deep breath." Nor did I like the idea of people covering my body with gunk, whether it be crushed pineapple, Dead Sea mud, or melted chocolate. I started writing about spas because I loved travel as a means of escape and insight. Entering a new culture is as dramatic as stepping inside a movie screen. Suddenly, one becomes part of a new world of flavors, colors, and customs. Every detail of life, from ordering breakfast to walking down the street, becomes an adventure. At its best, travel is not only a diversion from our everyday lives, but an intensification of life itself, enhancing our appreciation of the world around us, opening our minds to new perspectives.

During my first few spa trips, I realized spas are ideal places to deepen that shift in perspective. Many are in exotic locales and near sites rich in history. They also provide lots of time to sit still, reflect, and learn. My spa journeys have made me stronger, more confident, and less fearful. When I arrived at a small spa in British Columbia, I was afraid of horses; by the end of my stay, I was cantering through the meadow with the wind blowing through my hair. Later, I used the Equine Program at Miraval (see page 18) to explore my attitudes towards control, anger, and fear.

Linda and I have met people whose spa journeys have led them to change their careers, their boyfriends, even their religions. We've met others who used their spa experience to help them recover from illness or the death of a loved one, and in one case, a rape. These people turned to spas to help quiet the obsessive mental chatter that churns in the mind like a hamster wheel. And quieting the mental noise, or "monkey mind," as the Buddhists call it, allows new insights to enter in.

"Signs appear to those who look for them," wrote playwright August Strindberg. And spas are great places to look for those signs. One woman told me that as she was hiking during a spa journey, she realized how hard she was on herself. "We were on this muddy trail and I couldn't keep up with the group. I started putting all kinds of pressure on myself to catch up. Then I took a deep breath and I saw the mud as old negative habits that were pulling me down, and I realized that my concern about 'keeping up with the rest' was something that dogged me all the time. And then it came to me: *It's okay to go at my own pace. I should be kinder to myself.* Now when I start getting hard on myself, I remember my trip and stop."

The spas in this book have been chosen not only for the quality of their treatments, food, and amenities, but for their unique features and programs that allow visitors to glean life-changing revelations. The selection is diverse, for spa journeys can be as varied as any vacation experience. But there are basically two distinct types: one, known as a *destination spa*, focuses primarily on getting fit (only low-fat food is offered); the other is a *resort spa*, which offers the spa lifestyle as one of many options. But every spa listed in this book offers a host of activities beyond massages and facials. You can stroll the hills of Tuscany, climb a waterfall in a Hawaiian rain forest, or take a helicopter ride over the Canadian Rockies. More adventurous souls can go whitewater rafting, rock climbing, or mountain biking.

Of course, if you prefer, you can just sit by the pool all day, get a good massage... and look for signs that will bring you closer to the secrets inside yourself.

—Annette Foglino

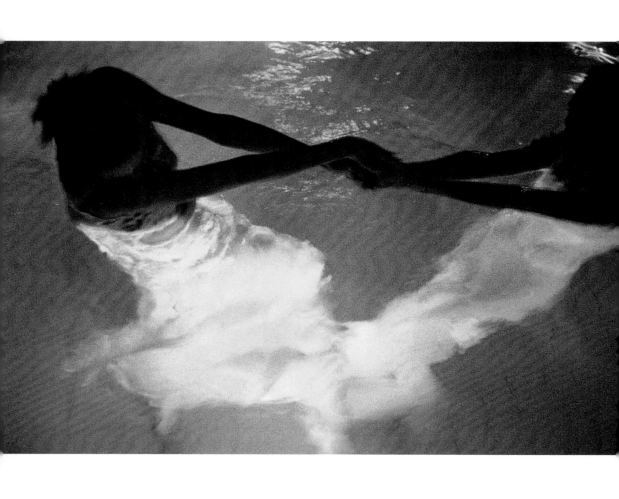

Spas have had a profound impact on my photography. At spas, I fell in love with the idea of capturing the image of what an epiphany, or shift in consciousness, might look like. I wanted to show the beauty, sensuality, and tranquility inherent in most spas—but not in an airbrushed way.

When I started shooting in treatment rooms, I had to use fast film and a slow shutter speed, because there wasn't much light. This caused a lot of movement and blur. This grainy, blurry quality felt right to me, as if I were capturing what it's like to go inside my subject's head. The filmmaker Wim Wenders once said, "the graininess of an image can have an interior life."

I continue to explore the interior life in my photography with more clean lines and space, and I've become more aware of using color to provide a feeling of well-being. I focus on just a hand on a horse with lots of sky behind, or the simple elegance of a few red pillows on a couch.

Photography is immensely healing as a form of self-expression. Some spas recognize this and offer photo classes; you can even make your own self-portraits as you evolve. Going through pictures of your former lives and unhappy situations, editing them, and restoring order with new images can rejuvenate your soul. The photography in this book is an invitation to explore art as transformation.

—LINDA TROELLER

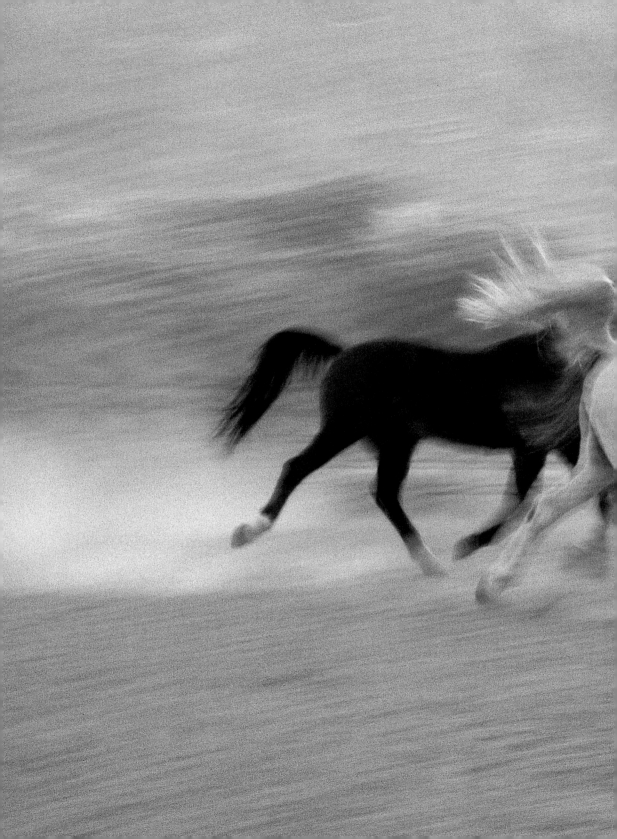

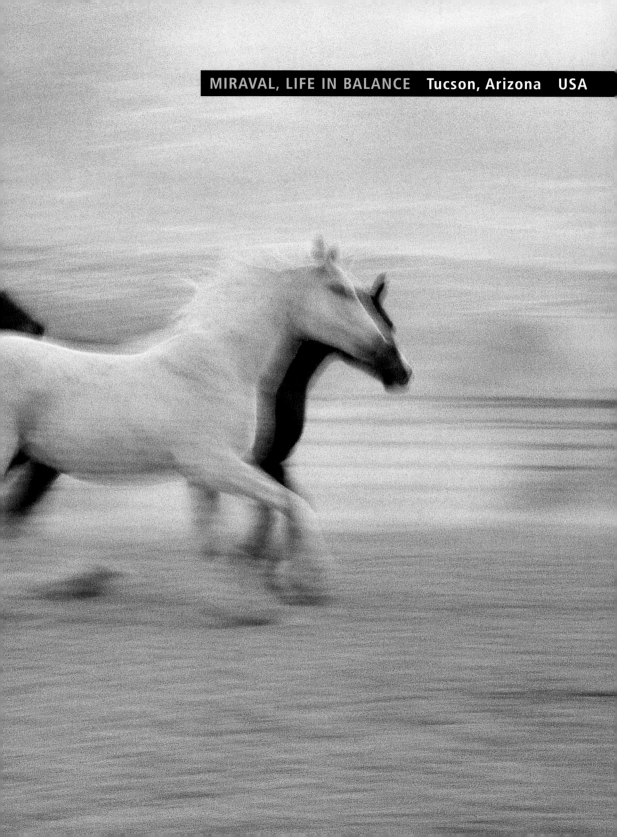

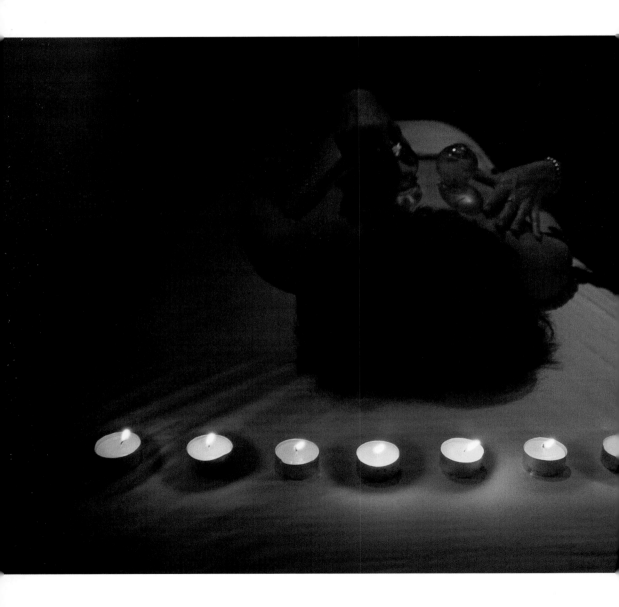

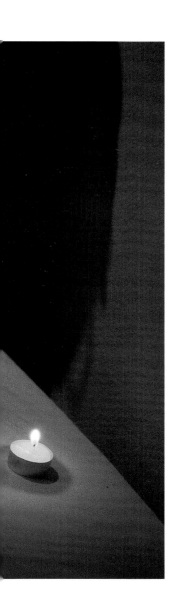

MIRAVAL, LIFE IN BALANCE, TUCSON

For many, a part of the Miraval experience is crying. In some respects, it could be described as the Barbara Walters spa experience ("It's okay to cwy, deah"), but in truth, it's more an Oprah kind of place. Don't let this scare you; the crying isn't about self-pity. It's meant to be cathartic and there are plenty of pleasant Dr. Phil–types to make you feel better. And it's hard to remain gloomy in such an enchanting desert atmosphere. Miraval is consistently rated one of the top spas in the United States.

Many of the guests are stressed-out New Yorkers, who come with the hope of slowing down and learning "mindfulness"—the "be-in-the-moment" philosophy that is this spa's trademark. But for the most part visitors are a diverse group, from all walks of life, and include single men, still a rarity at most spas. Mike Doyle, a thirty-year-old car salesman from Long Island, NY, decided to visit after he quit his job and wasn't sure what he would do next. "I was in line at the supermarket feeling really burned out when I saw Oprah's magazine," he says. "The cover read 'Top Ten Ways to De-stress,' or something to that effect. Miraval was mentioned, so I reserved a flight to Tucson the next day."

Miraval is an excellent place to visit when you're at a crossroads in life. A hazy, purple mountain range is the perfect backdrop for self-reflection. And Miraval offers innovative classes and meditation techniques for exploring a new perspective in life. Try Quantum Leap, where participants climb a twenty-five-foot pole while a group of peers hold the ropes below. Or participate in a more sedentary endeavor like a Holographic Memory session, which begins with you focusing on any bodily pain you may have, then picturing a scene from your past; in so doing you utilize visualization to "reframe" the memory in order to make it a more positive one.

At Miraval, even the horses are transformed into New Age healers. The popular Equine Program was developed by psychologist Wyatt Webb, who once worked as a rehab counselor at Sierra Tucson, a clinic specializing in addiction (and owned by Miraval). A former country musician, Wyatt sports a shaggy, gray beard and a down-to-earth, aw-shucks-I've-been-around demeanor that make him the perfect cowboy shrink. He's affectionately known as "Wyatt" to just about anyone who has ever completed the Equine Program. The premise of the program is that horses, sensitive creatures finely tuned to their surroundings, can help us to become more self-aware, as they mirror our emotions.

Wyatt discovered the healing power of horses while working with troubled teenagers in the late 1980s. "These kids were angry, but they would often let their guard down with the horses," he says. "It was much easier to deal with their issues through the use of a horse." In 1995, Wyatt decided to see if adults would respond the same way.

THIS SPA IS FOR YOU IF you love both spiritual retreats and luxurious pampering.

THIS SPA IS NOT FOR YOU IF touchy-feely, New Age rhetoric nauseates you.

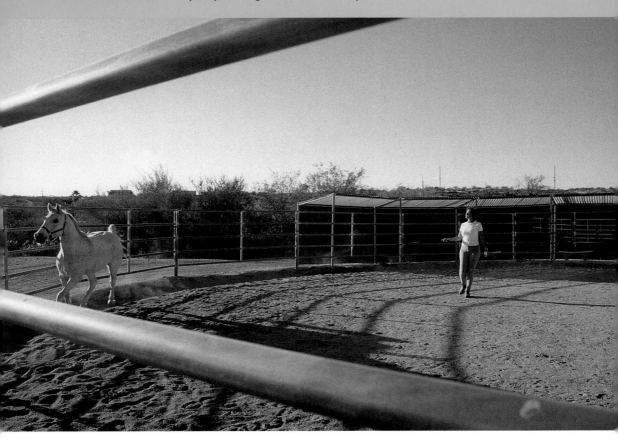

PRICE $$$$$

ROOMS 106
A notch above basic, clean & pleasant.

FOOD
The main dining room is famous for its all-you-can-eat spa buffet. Breakfast and lunches are a smorgasbord of low-fat culinary creativity. Dinner includes innovative gourmet meals with a Southwestern flourish (e.g. red chili, yellow corn, and turkey in mole sauce).

OUTSTANDING TREATMENTS
Hot Stone Massage; Sagebrush Friction (a massage that improves circulation and relieves muscle soreness—sagebrush is an herb traditionally used by Native Americans for rheumatism); Moxibustion Acupuncture (uses heat on acupuncture points).

ACTIVITIES
Horseback Riding; Golf (nearby); Tennis; and Hiking.

CLASSES
Sunset and Horseplay Photography; Equine Experience; Quantum Leap; Wall Climbing; Mindful Decision-Making; Mindful Relationships; Mindful Eating; Water Conditioning; Star Gazing; Chi Kung; Pilates; and Yoga.

GETTING THERE
A half-hour's drive from Tucson airport.

ADDRESS
5000 East Via Estancia Miraval Catalina, AZ 85739

T 800-232-3969   **F** 520-825-5163   **E** miraval@lifeinbalance.com   **W** www.miravalresort.com

Indeed they did. The Equine Program is a huge draw at Miraval. Surprisingly, the program doesn't involve getting on a horse. First, one grooms the animal, brushing it and cleaning its hooves. Then, participants get the horse to walk, trot, and gallop around a large ring. As you do all of this, Wyatt can pinpoint ways you may sabotage yourself in your life in general. "You can tell a lot about someone by how they interact with a horse," says Wyatt, whose recent book is called, *It's Not about the Horse: It's about Us, Seeing How the Stories We Create Shape Our Lives*. "If people have fear issues, for example, they're going to be raised around a 1,200 pound animal."

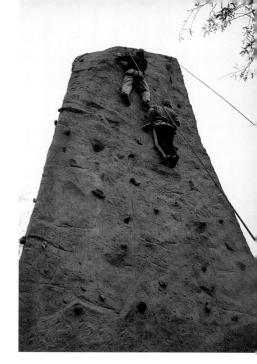

Much information is revealed during the hoof cleaning. "Stressed-out, aggressive people will try to push the horse into cooperating—it never occurs to them to ask for help," says Wyatt. "Once they realize they can ask for help, a new world opens up to them."

I definitely fell into the "stressed-out, aggressive" category, but I wasn't about to bully a huge animal. I asked for help right away, but I still couldn't get the horse to lift its hoof. "What are you feeling?" Wyatt asked me.

"Anger," I replied.

"Anger at whom?" asked Wyatt.

"The horse. Me."

"Well, if you're angry at the horse, you're wasting your time. He's just an animal that doesn't know you. Why are you angry at yourself?"

"Because I should be able to do this," I replied, looking around and seeing others already cleaning their third hoof.

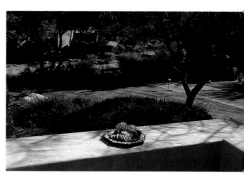

"And what if you can't?"

That was the question. In about ten minutes, Wyatt was able to identify one of my major issues: When I get angry I turn the anger in on myself. Wyatt encouraged me to acknowledge my anger and use it to my advantage. I took a deep breath, walked up to the horse again, and it lifted its hoof for me.

Far deeper issues emerge for others. One woman took part in the program every day for over a week to confront fear and other emotions after being raped years before. "I had been numb for a long time," she said. "It may sound strange, but working with the horses—and connecting with a creature so overpowering—helped me to reclaim myself."

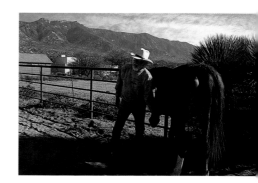

Mike from Long Island confronted his issues by trying to persuade the horse to move in a circle around him. It's euphoric to control such a huge animal with just your movements; you're in sync with it. If you know what you're doing, one breath will slow the horse down or even bring him to a stop. Turn your back to him with the right attitude, and he will come over and nuzzle you like a dog. Mike wanted his horse to slow down, but it took off at a gallop. "That's why I'm here," he later told me, "to learn to slow down."

While the Equine Program is the main attraction, it is quite possible to enjoy Miraval without ever laying eyes on a horse. With the huge array of self-discovery courses offered, you'll still come away enlightened—even through the tears.

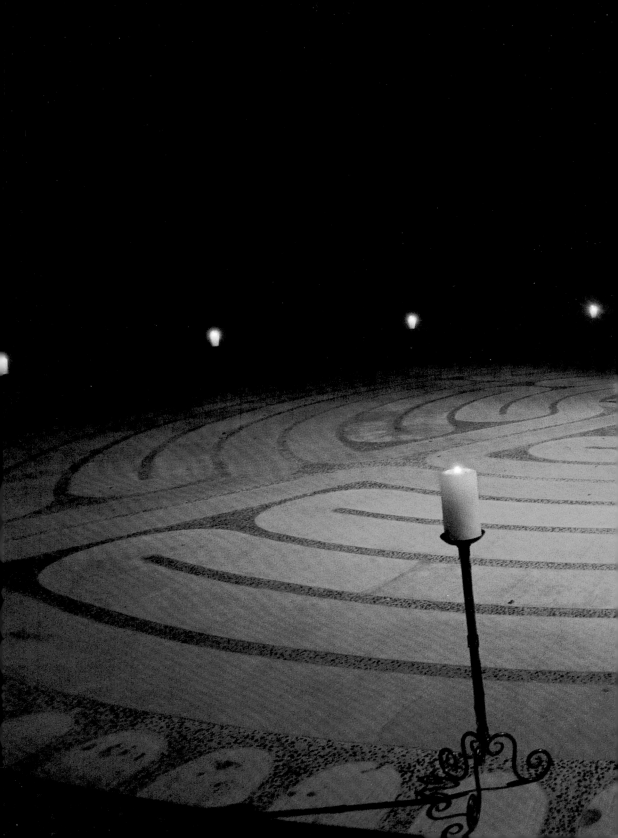

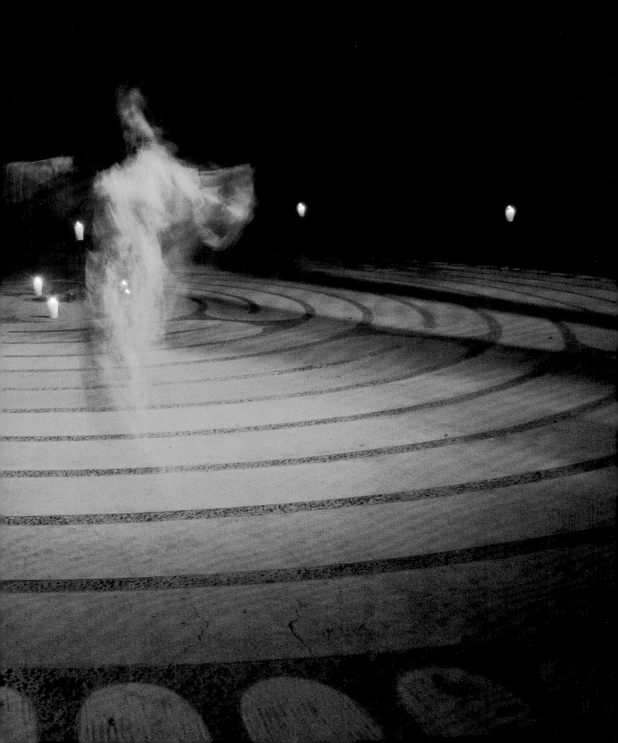

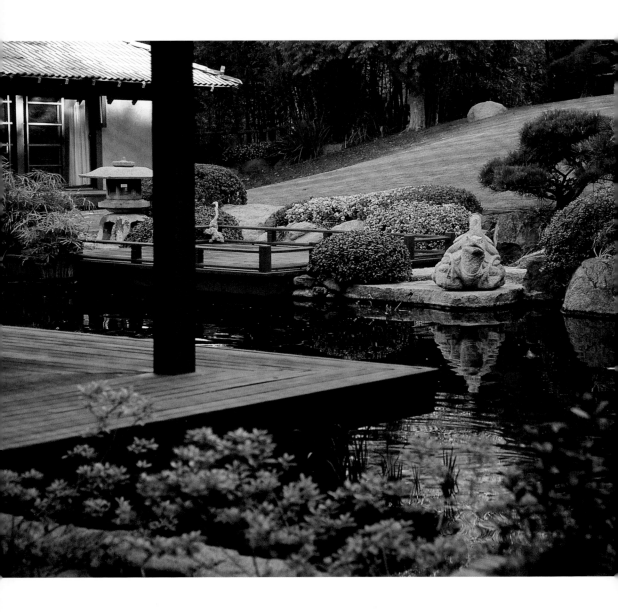

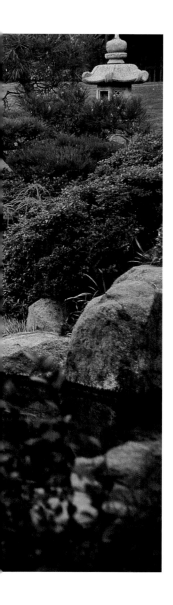

THE GOLDEN DOOR, ESCONDIDO

The entrance to the Golden Door is actually polished brass, but once you pass through it, there's no mistaking the Midas glow shimmering throughout the entire spa. Designed to resemble a Japanese *honjin*, or hot springs inn, it is most definitely Zen California-style, featuring a koi-filled lake and meditation gardens. Beyond the "golden" gate, you'll find the highest level of pampering in a world so serene and comforting, it's like having an indulgent mother, an English butler, and a personal trainer attending to your every need. You won't care if the doors ever open again.

With a staff-to-guest ratio of four-to-one, you are alternately coddled and coaxed into pursuing a healthier lifestyle. Each week, forty guests arrive on Sunday and leave the following Saturday. Only female guests are in residence for that time, but the spa offers coed visits intermittently.

The Golden Door opened in 1958, created by Deborah Szekely as a sister-spa to Rancho La Puerta, the health resort she had started with her husband in Mexico eighteen years earlier (see page 174). Hollywood actors and other celebrities were continuously emerging from Rancho looking slimmer and feeling healthier. They wanted a similar place closer to home. "We were in what was called the 'Golden Age' of motion pictures," says Szekely. "The directors and performers who loved going to the Ranch watched it evolve from a small primitive fitness-camp to a large rustic resort—but they wanted more privacy and intimacy."

The Golden Door still attracts its share of the Hollywood elite, CEOs, and ladies-who-lunch, and if you're willing to splurge, you might find yourself rubbing elbows and sharing yoga tips with them over an impeccable gourmet meal. Such a meal will consist of some of the freshest and most delicious food you've ever tasted, such as grilled duck breast in a peanut-ginger sauce, Alaskan crab on a bed of tender greens, or herb-encrusted rack of venison. (The Door set the standard for haute cuisine spa food, and the fare is still as good as it gets—fresh fish is flown in daily.) As at many destination spas, guests are encouraged to wear (and are provided with) shorts, T-shirts, and sweat suits, and this is a great equalizer. A stylish uniform of the Japanese *yukata*, a cotton robe, also adds to the bonding experience.

Or instead of bonding, you can just have dinner in your room. Most rooms are spare with elegant touches, such as tatami floors, shoji screens, fresh flowers, and small, private outdoor gardens. Each morning, breakfast is delivered accompanied by a paper fan on which is handwritten a Zen poem and a schedule of activities. These activities are selected by your personal trainer, and are based upon an assessment made after your initial physical exam.

The morning usually includes the more rigorous pursuits, from hiking to tap dancing, from weight-training to water aerobics. Guests with physical challenges will find themselves well accommodated by their trainer. "I could not

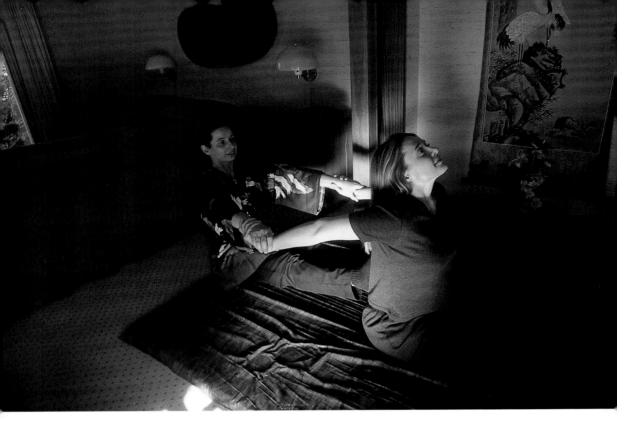

PRICE $$$$$

ROOMS 40
Elegantly appointed.

FOOD
Exceptional and creative low-fat gourmet. Use of fresh and organic produce. No red meat or alcohol. Desserts range from chocolate Mexican flan to apple cranberry strudel.

T 760-744-5777

OUTSTANDING TREATMENTS
Warm Honey Wrap with an Orange Blossom Milk Soak; Kiatsu (healing water massage); and Oxygen Facial Mask.

ACTIVITIES
Walking the labyrinth; Getting a makeover; and Hiking. Lectures on everything from health to the art of bonsai.

F 760-471-2393

CLASSES
A wide array: Archery; Fencing; Cooking; Poetry; Feldenkrais (body manipulation to reprogram the nervous system); Salsa; NIA (nonimpact aerobics, combining martial arts and dance); Country Dancing; Cardioboxing; Tai Chi; Pilates; and Yoga.

E gdres@adnc.com

NEARBY ATTRACTIONS
San Diego beaches; the town of La Jolla; Sea World; Wild Animal Park; Tijuana, Mexico.

GETTING THERE
A 45-minute drive from San Diego airport.

ADDRESS
PO Box 463077
Escondido, CA 92046-3077

W www.goldendoor.com

THIS SPA IS FOR YOU IF you want the ultimate in self-reflection and pampering.
THIS SPA IS NOT FOR YOU IF you have a small budget.

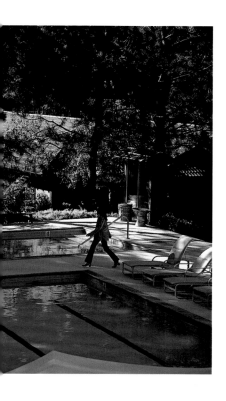

get my heart rate up to where it was supposed to be," says Linda Troeller, this book's photographer. "Signe, the trainer, was very creative without putting too much pressure on me. She showed me how to move my arms in a way that didn't hurt and helped me exert myself more. At the end of my stay, I had to walk around a huge field. I didn't think I could make it, but with her help, I did."

In the afternoon, you're free to try things you've probably never done before, such as writing haiku poetry, fencing, archery, and even something called "natural vision enhancement," a series of eye exercises practiced by yogis. Or opt for the more familiar and have a facial, a manicure, or a massage—all part of the daily routine. Indeed, at the end of the day, a masseuse will come to your room, put on some soothing music, and knead and coax your muscles into the mood for peaceful slumber.

Along with all the pampering and physical conditioning, the Golden Door offers exercises and tools for self-reflection. This spa is one of the first to have installed a walking labyrinth on the grounds. Guests are encouraged to walk the winding path to its center and back out again. Labyrinths are not mazes; they don't have dead ends, but they circle around and wind back to the center. In the Middle Ages, walking a labyrinth was believed to have been a substitute for making the pilgrimage to Jerusalem.

In its way, the Golden Door presents walking the labyrinth as a pilgrimage to oneself. Some may find walking the circle somewhat tedious. I would much prefer strolling a wooded path, but others find it an effective way to focus. The spa has devised a labyrinth ritual as well: You write down on a piece of paper something you want to change about yourself or your life, walk to the center of the labyrinth, and deposit the paper into a clay pot to be burned. One guest reported that this rite introduced her to the concept of meditation. "I've never kept still for anything in my life, except sleep," she says. "The idea of moving with no destination in mind— no *outward* destination, I mean—was so foreign to me. But walking the labyrinth made me realize that I don't always have to be going somewhere, physically, in order to make positive changes in my life. I need more self-awareness, and meditation is a great way to get it."

Some guests, like Linda, were trying to leave their sadness over a loved-one behind. "My mother had died over a year before, and I wanted to replace my feelings of grief with a sense of having her with me as a friend with whom I could still talk," she says. "As I walked the labyrinth, I noticed how hard it was to stay within the borders. I saw it as a metaphor for my life, especially with its twists and turns, and what it takes to get to a healthier place. When I got to the center, I deposited the tiny note in the clay pot, where it went up in flames. I viewed this as my intention to move on and cherish my new relationship with her."

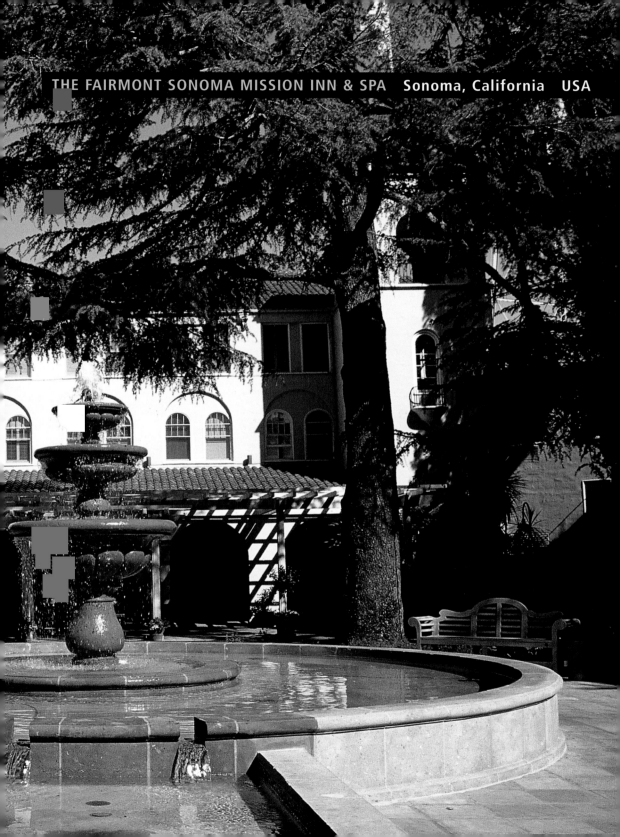

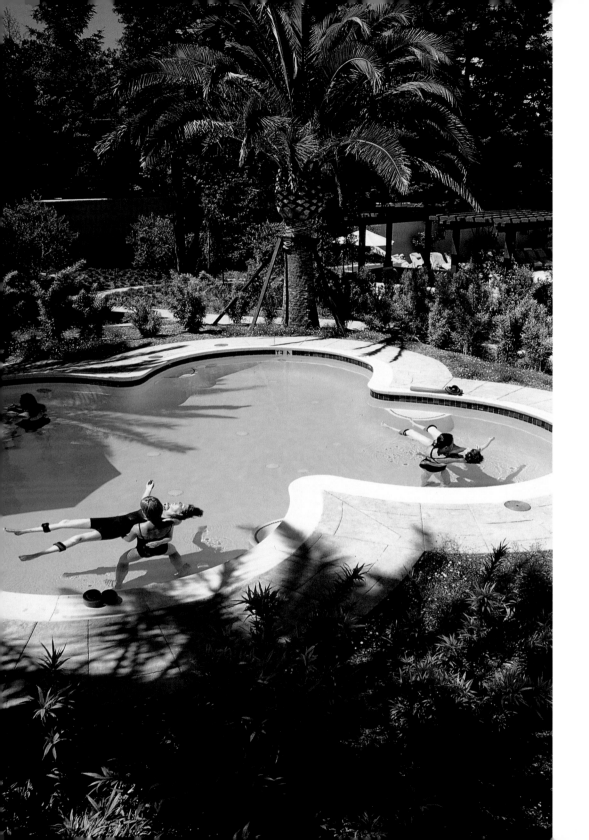

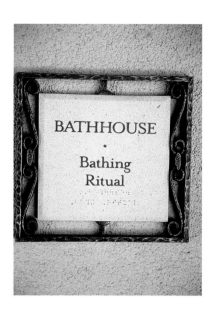

THE FAIRMONT SONOMA MISSION INN & SPA, SONOMA

Wine, water, and roses. Used properly, the combination creates the perfect romance, and all are utilized to perfection here. In the heart of the lush California wine country, a bath filled with thermal waters and rose petals coupled with a wood-burning fireplace made this one of the most romantic places I've ever been to—and I was here by myself.

The resort has a rich history as a utopian retreat. Hundreds of years ago Native Americans, who believed in the curative and sensual power of mineral waters, considered this site to be sacred because of its natural thermal springs. A San Francisco doctor bought the land in 1840, and developed it into a health resort. Fifty years later enterprising Englishman Captain H. E. Boyes expanded the place into a luxury resort, where the wealthy could "take the waters" in, European style. In the early 1920s, the Boyes Springs Hotel advertised such amenities as electricity and running water, as well as "moving pictures, competent masseurs and masseuses, and the largest mineral water swimming tank in the world."

Today, after several renovations, the inn, now a pretty, pink mission-style building, has plenty of thermal water to go around, and massage therapists who are more than merely "competent." Though it can no longer boast the "largest mineral water swimming tank in the world," the spa does have a spectacular Roman-bath motif dominating its 40,000 square-feet. Grand columns and pastel murals provide a backdrop to two pools of mineral water, one pool heated to 98 degrees, the other to 102 degrees. The spa has devised a "bathing ritual" similar to that of the ancient Romans. You start the ritual in warm water and then proceed to the hotter soak. Next it's on to a cool plunge beneath giant massaging showerheads, finishing with an herbal steam or sauna. I encourage anyone receiving a treatment to take advantage of the bathing ritual, which is free of charge. (There is a $35 fee without a treatment.)

For further water-indulgence, try a *Watsu* treatment in the outdoor pool. The massage therapist cradles you like a baby, and then stretches you, sometimes swirling you around as in an aquatic ballet. It's intimate, yet at the same time the therapist manages to keep a respectful distance.

The wine-and-water theme reaches a crescendo with the Wine Country *Kur* treatment. It begins with a soak in water mixed with grapeseeds, and finishes with a grapeseed-oil scrub, which exfoliates and moisturizes the skin. Grapes, of course, are an excellent source of antioxidants—even in wine.

Lest you feel you're drowning in water treatments, there's plenty to do in between, from bicycling through the wine country (with a few stops for tasting along the way) to hiking and hot-air ballooning. At the end of the day, if you want to step back into the water, several rooms have a giant tub with room for two, and a view of the fireplace. Order a bottle of wine from the resort's award-winning selection and let the romance begin.

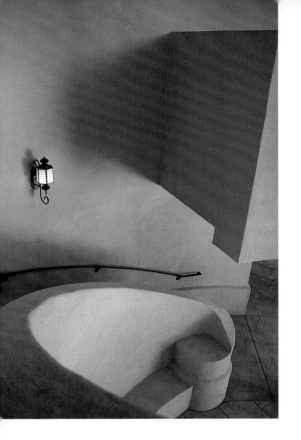

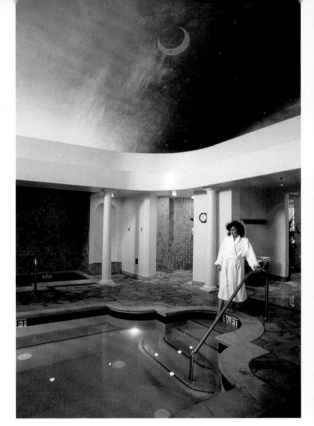

THIS SPA IS FOR YOU IF you want a romantic getaway and you love wine, water, and food.

THIS SPA IS NOT FOR YOU IF you've just broken up with someone.

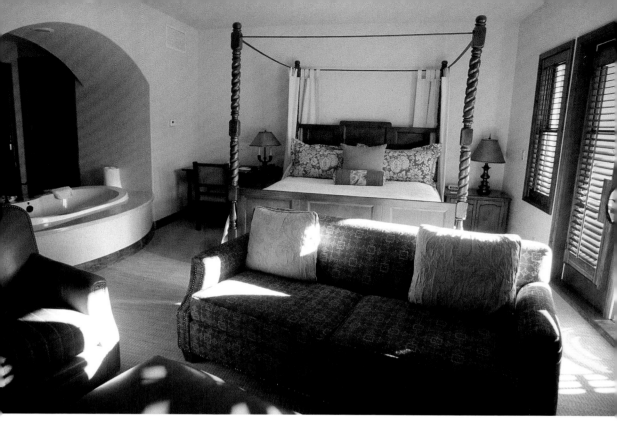

PRICE $$$

ROOMS 223
Elegantly appointed.
Some with beamed
ceilings, fluffy white
comforters, and mission-
style decor. Mission suites
have in-room whirlpool
baths with a view of a
wood-burning fireplace.

FOOD
Two restaurants: one
casual and one gourmet.
The casual restaurant is
called **BIG 3 DINER**, but it's
not really a diner. It's

West Coast elegant with
excellent California
cuisine, offering salads
made from fresh local
ingredients. The gourmet
restaurant is described as
"progressive wine-country
cuisine," which includes
foie gras, duck, and lamb.
A chef's tasting menu is
also available.

**OUTSTANDING
TREATMENTS**
The Couples King Bath
(a tub for two of mineral
water and rose petals,
followed by a massage);

the Wine Country Kur
(a soak and then a scrub
with a grapeseed
concoction of body polish
and moisturizer); Watsu
(water massage) in a
scenic outdoor pool.

ACTIVITIES
18-hole Golf Course;
Horseback Riding; Hiking;
Tennis; Biking; and
Hot-Air Ballooning.

CLASSES
Cardio; Bodybuilding;
Aqua-Aerobics; and Yoga.

NEARBY ATTRACTIONS
The home of writer Jack
London (of *The Call of the
Wild* fame), preserved in
an 800-acre state park.

GETTING THERE
A 90-minute drive from
San Francisco airport.

ADDRESS
Sonoma Mission Inn & Spa
PO Box 1447
Sonoma, CA 95476-1447

T 707-938-9000   **F** 707-938-4250   **E** smi.reservations@fairmont.com   **W** www.fairmont.com

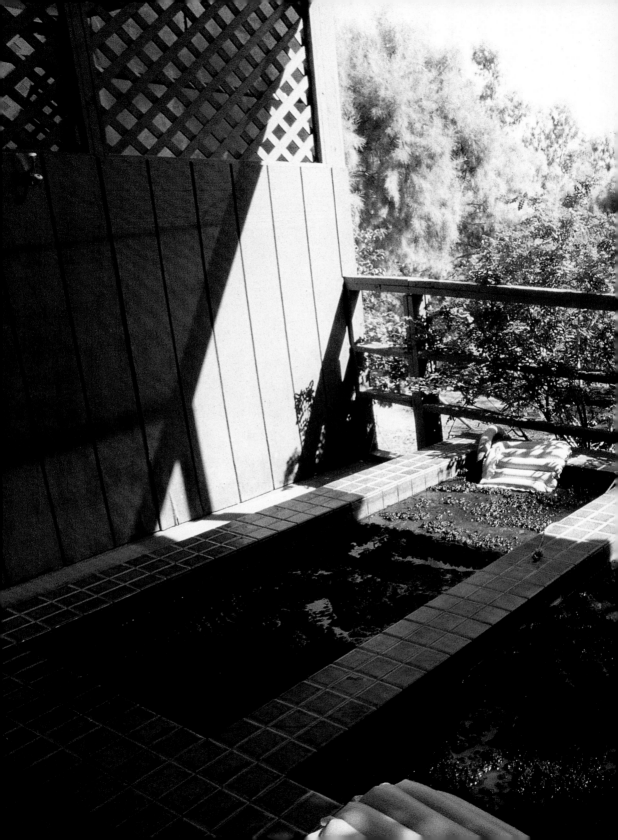

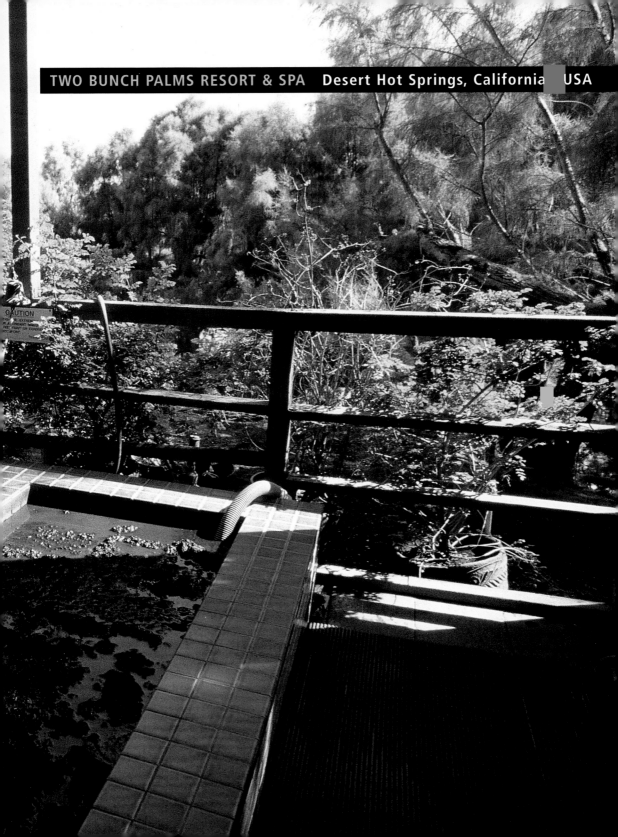

CAUTION

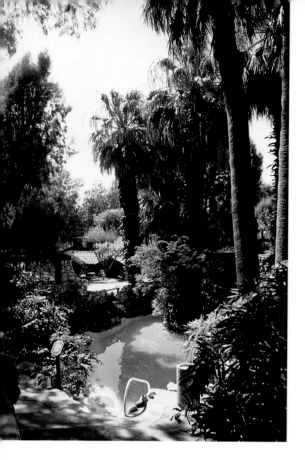

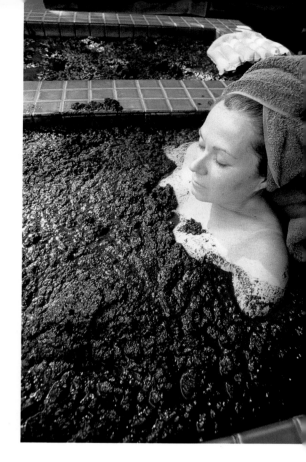

PRICE $$$–$$$$
($$$ weekday specials)

ROOMS 45
Run the gamut
from basic, clean &
pleasant to elegantly
appointed.

FOOD
The main restaurant serves
California cuisine that
includes quite a few
fattening treats, such as
baked brie with a fruit
plate. But of course, there
is enough low-fat fare to
go around.

**OUTSTANDING
TREATMENTS**
Color Therapy; Watsu; and
Mud Baths.

CLASSES
Yoga by the lake.

NEARBY ATTRACTIONS
Palm Springs.

GETTING THERE
A 20-minute drive from
Palm Springs airport.

ADDRESS
67-425 Two Bunch
Palms Trail
Desert Hot Springs, CA
92240

T 760-329-8791   **F** 760-329-1317   **E** whiteowl@twobunchpalms.com   **W** www.twobunchpalms.com

THIS SPA IS FOR YOU IF you want to escape from civilization and decompress.

THIS SPA IS NOT FOR YOU IF you want to start a new fitness regimen, enjoy organized activities, or expect snappy
service from hotel staff.

TWO BUNCH PALMS RESORT & SPA, DESERT HOT SPRINGS

Millions of years ago, the desert surrounding Palm Springs was covered by water, and the landscape still resembles the ocean bottom. For miles around, all you can see is clay-colored sand, tumbleweeds, and sagebrush, with an occasional fast-food wrapper bumping along in the wind. Two Bunch Palms, about ten miles from Palm Springs, is off the beaten path, as it was when Al Capone supposedly used it as a hideaway from the Feds. It's tucked away on a desert road in a secluded location, which is one reason why it is a favored spot for Hollywood's elite seeking a quick escape from Los Angeles.

As you drive past the guard at the gate, don't expect to be overwhelmed by uniformed attendants, lavish potted plants, and grand archways. Everyone, no matter how famous, wheels their own luggage to their rooms, some of which seem to be frozen in the 1970s. Suites are outfitted with Spanish orange tiles, wicker dining tables, and La-Z-Boy-type furniture. (Mel Gibson stayed in one suite decorated with an iridescent velvet painting of an eerie-looking guru, although I'm told the decor has been updated with a more contemporary collection of mirrors.) There is also a large guest house high on a hill offering spectacular views, outdoor hot tubs, and fireplaces—the scene of many a celebrity pajama party. Older rooms, though decorated with antiques, have a hodgepodge and decidedly funky vibe, reminiscent of the flower children who flocked here in the sixties.

The mineral waters continue to be a major draw. The stone-lined grotto pool is a veritable oasis, filled with thermal water, surrounded by lush vegetation, and shaded by palm trees; one tree rises from a tiny island in the pool itself. The water originates from a geological fault and bubbles up at a temperature of 140 degrees Fahrenheit; it is cooled to body temperature before it flows into the pool. (In one section the water temperature is kept at 104 degrees for those who can take it.) Unlike many thermal springs, this water has no sulfurous odor, and because it's constantly moving it's more likely to be free of bacteria.

Guests float face up, just drifting and listening to the quiet. Signs are posted everywhere requesting that everyone keep their voices down. Cell phones are regarded with hostility. Many water-lovers stay immersed all afternoon while reading a book or a screenplay. This is not a place to overtax oneself: there is no exercise equipment. It's all about settling oneself into nature, looking up at a canopy of tamarisk trees while luxuriating in the pool, as hummingbirds zip and swoop overhead. Boisterous ravens as large as baby seals and clever-looking bunnies dart and hop about the lawn.

The spa boasts a huge selection of innovative treatments. These include acupressure therapy; chakra color therapy, which involves deep-breathing in an octagon-shaped room with stained-glass windows; and *Watsu*, an incredibly serene form of water massage. An open cabana offers baths of mud mixed with the thermal waters. The mud, which looks like molten lumps of coal combined with dirt and straw, may appear unappealing to some. In the movie *The Player*, actor Tim Robbins eases himself into these baths with such aplomb, he makes it look fun. But I found climbing in rather gross—both a grainy and a slimy experience. But once I could ignore the viscosity, the mud's heavy warmth felt like a cozy blanket.

Most visitors to Two Bunch are happy to surrender to unstructured days, ready to do nothing but float. Occasionally, however, some find it a bit slow, as Anna Nicole Smith did during one of her stays. Anna Nicole reportedly got so antsy that she made friends with some of the busboys, and they all drove into town to eat and party, and party and eat.

Two Bunch will appeal to those for whom nightlife means lolling in a twenty-four-hour mineral pool. At midnight, try floating silently, gazing up at the diamond stars in the shimmering desert sky, and listen as a coyote cries in the distance.

MANDARIN ORIENTAL Miami, Florida USA

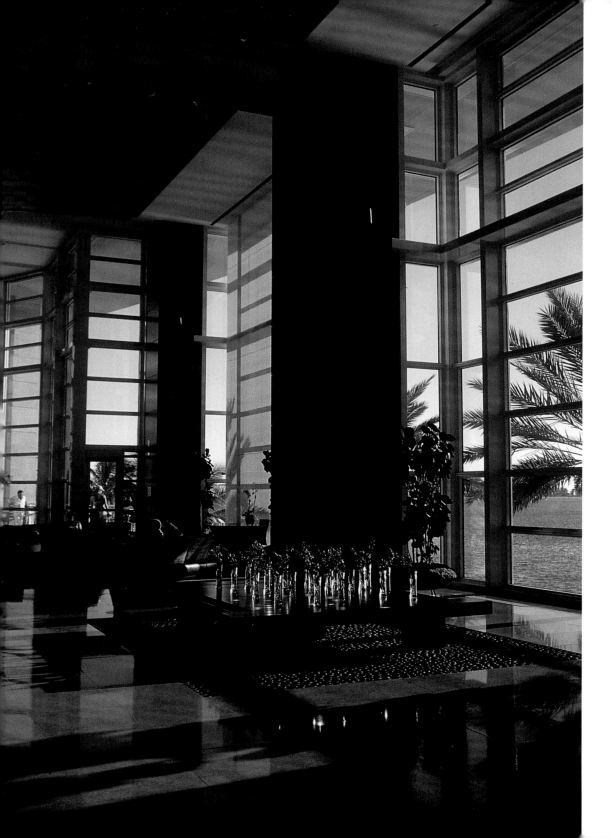

MANDARIN ORIENTAL, MIAMI

If you're looking for an island of peace amid the heat and sizzling bustle of Miami, here is your refuge. It is a rare place where the lobby is almost as relaxing as the spa. Upon entering, you are greeted with tiny, flower-filled glass vases set on a low table, the water in each reflecting the rippling waters of Biscayne Bay outside—a sort of Zen sculpture that cues body and mind to decompress. One look at the art deco lobby, its trees and smooth black rocks, and the tension melts off your back.

Asian-themed rooms are similarly soothing. Cream-colored walls and down comforters complement dark Oriental furniture, bamboo, and orchids. The Mandarin chain is known for its luxury and clean elegance, reflected in the company logo, a simple, splayed gold fan. Some rooms open onto a marble bath area, allowing a soak in the tub while looking out at the bay and Miami skyline. They're the kind of rooms where one could stay all day, losing track of time.

The spa has its own special way of helping you to lose track, with its signature treatment, ironically named the Time Ritual, which takes place in one of six spa suites. Almost as large as a regular hotel room, with CD players, phones, and showers, the pink marble suites are a symphony of spa luxury, with candles, tiny bowls of aromatherapy herbs, and floor-to-ceiling windows that have a view of the bay. Orchids, practically an Asian spa symbol, are omnipresent, placed on towels, slippers, and massage tables.

The word "pamper" is overused in the spa world, but it's almost impossible to overuse it here. The moment you sit down with your ritual therapist, you are treated like royalty. And if you're squeamish about people fussing over you, it might even feel embarrassing. My therapist, Carlos, a gentle bear of a man from Puerto Rico, welcomes me by clasping one of my hands in his as he guides me toward a chair (resembling a tiny throne), next to which is a bowl of water scented with oils and flower petals. He kneels and takes my foot, rubs it with oil, and asks a few general questions about my likes and dislikes, thereby determining my body type. My type, based on the Indian Ayurvedic system, indicates which oils and treatments are appropriate for me.

One would think that after years of writing about spas I'd be accustomed to pampering, but when Carlos plunges my foot into the bowl of flower petals I feel a little self-conscious about having someone washing my feet. Spa novices and those who don't like being fussed over take note: *Get over it.* As Carlos kneads and glides the oil over my feet, I sip ginger tea and listen as he tells me about his time as a physical therapist in a mental hospital. He seems to have the perfect calm demeanor for the job (the mental hospital and the spa).

Next it's onto the table where I'm covered in a gritty apricot scrub (a little rough, but fragrant) before being cleaned off with warm linens. Massaging me, Carlos dribbles heated oil over me and it feels as if the drops are dancing on my skin. I get into the rhythm of warm linens, streams of oil, and hands on my body. At some point, creams and lotions are massaged into my face by the firm flurry of Carlos' fingers before I succumb to a scalp massage. The echo of tiny brass cymbals signals the ritual is over.

The whole thing lasted two hours, and at $260 is not cheap. But for the ultimate splurge, it's worth it. For more money, you can book more time and continue to customize your treatment. The spa has seventeen additional ordinary, non-suite treatment rooms, where you can book individual therapies.

As I floated off the table, I wondered if I had experienced pampering overload. But then I realized there is no such thing. Especially not here.

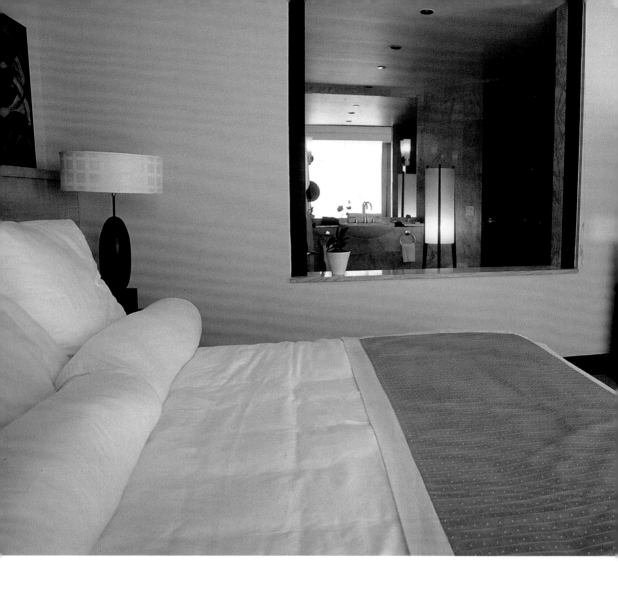

THIS SPA IS FOR YOU IF you want serene luxury in Miami.

THIS SPA IS NOT FOR YOU IF you want to be right in the heart of the action in South Beach.

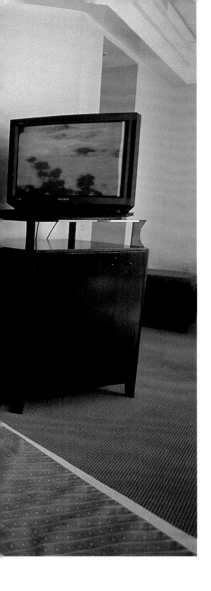

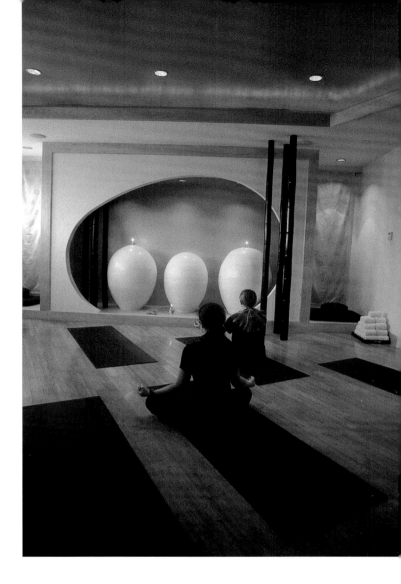

PRICE $$$$$

ROOMS 329
Sumptuous and luxurious.

FOOD
CAFÉ SAMBAL has delicious
sushi and a wonderful
low-fat chicken with a
glass noodle salad. **AZUL** is
the more upscale choice,
serving gourmet Asian

selections. Both have
spectacular views of
Biscayne Bay and the
Miami skyline.

**OUTSTANDING
TREATMENTS**
The Time Ritual (see text);
Balinese Synchronized
Massage (stretching and
rolling movements using
long deep strokes);

Purified Hot Linen Wrap;
and Couples Massage.

CLASSES
Yoga; Pilates; Tai Chi; and
Belly Dancing.

NEARBY ATTRACTIONS
Miami's art deco
architecture and the sun,
sand, and sizzle of
South Beach.

GETTING THERE
A 20-minute drive from
Miami airport.

ADDRESS
500 Brickell Key Drive
Miami, FL 33131

T 305-913-8288   **F** 305-913-8300   **E** momia-reservations@mogh.com   **W** www.mandarinoriental.com

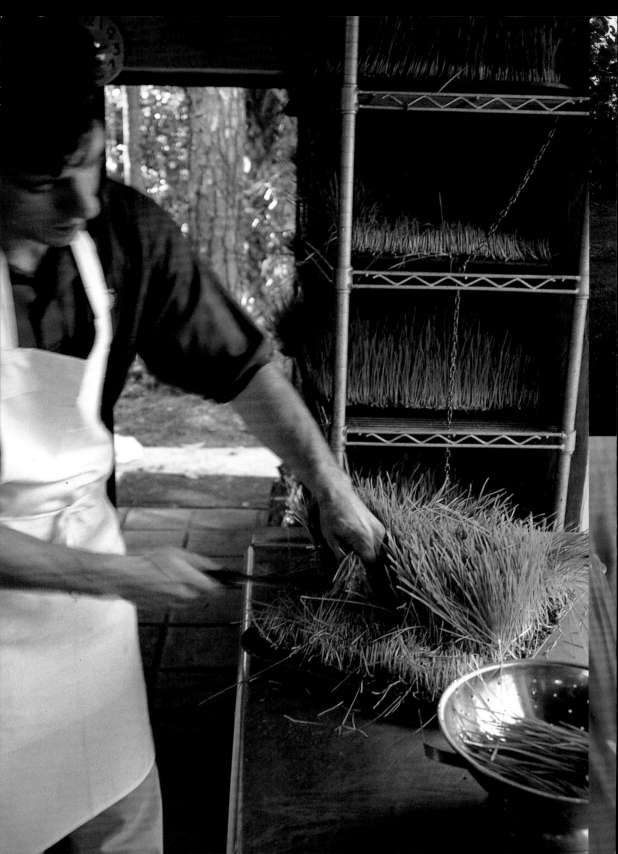

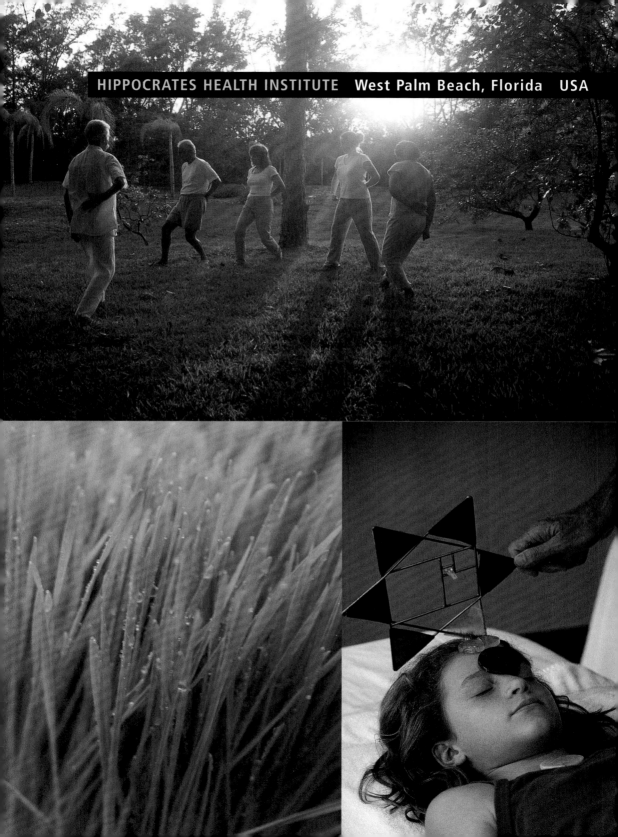

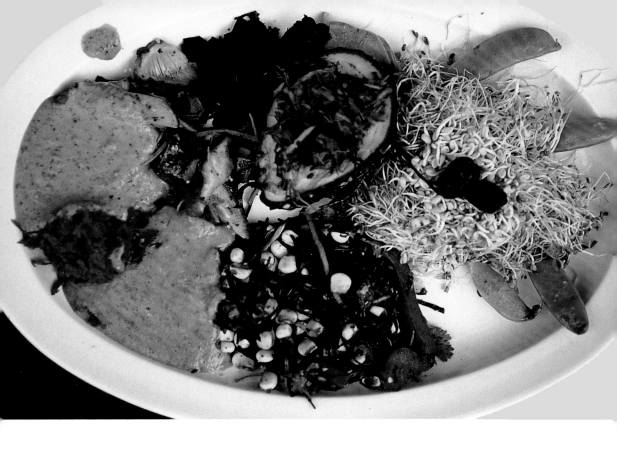

PRICE $$–$$$

ROOMS 29
From elegantly appointed suites to basic, clean & pleasant rooms.

FOOD
A buffet of fresh and raw vegetables, with more kinds of sprouts than you ever imagined.

OUTSTANDING TREATMENTS
Pain alleviation is a specialty. The Dia-Pulse machine addresses pain by heating up afflicted areas with electromagnetic heat. Laser-Frequency treatments are also available. Other treatments include Myofacial Release (connective tissue massage); Lymphatic Massage; and Scalp Massage.

ACTIVITIES
Health Lectures in outdoor pavilion; Field trips to nearby Japanese gardens; Organized walks.

CLASSES
Yoga; Tai Chi; Chi Kung; and Pilates.

NEARBY ATTRACTIONS
Dog track and Lion Country Safari.

GETTING THERE
A 15-minute drive from West Palm Beach airport.

ADDRESS
1443 Palmdale Court
West Palm Beach, FL 33411

T 800-842-2125   **F** 561-471-9464   **E** reservations@hippocratesinst.com   **W** www.hippocratesinst.com

THIS SPA IS FOR YOU IF you have serious health issues and want a strict detox program.
THIS SPA IS NOT FOR YOU IF your goal is strictly relaxation and luxury.

HIPPOCRATES HEALTH INSTITUTE, WEST PALM BEACH

Past the tinkling Spanish-tiled fountains, through the color-splashed tropical gardens, you come to the entrance of Hippocrates Health Institute. The South Florida air is warm and damp, and the sunny courtyard is reminiscent of a fun-loving Mexican resort. But despite all appearances, this is no place for a fiesta.

It's a place for serious healing. The main philosophy here is based on a well-known maxim of Hippocrates, the Greek philosopher and father of modern medicine: "Let the food be the medicine and the medicine be the food."

A brass gong along a winding path leading to the dining room summons guests to their daily medicine. The institute espouses a regimen of "live food," meaning 80 percent of the diet is uncooked fruits and vegetables. The program, founded in 1963 by a woman named Ann Wigmore, operates on the theory that cooking food destroys many important nutrients and enzymes required by the body to help repair itself. Uncooked foods and a positive attitude, Wigmore argued, can do wonders.

Lunch and dinner in the cozy main dining room is a buffet smorgasbord of sprouts, dried seaweed, salad, beans, nuts, peppers, tomatoes, and avocados. Warm soups are an indulgence only occasionally served. No dairy allowed.

Not far from the dining room is one of the main attractions of Hippocrates: the wheatgrass cottage, where rows of potted green squares smelling of dew wait to be squeezed into juice. Wheatgrass, full of potent enzymes, is believed to improve circulation and strengthen the immune system. Wheatgrass poultices are applied externally as well to treat infection or skin ailments.

The radical diet required by a stay at Hippocrates (many guests also receive colonics) causes some to feel worse before they feel better. But many who see the program through to its end report a spiritual, as well as a physical, rejuvenation. According to nutritionist Brian Clement, a disciple of Wigmore and now director of Hippocrates, the body retains toxins not just from the food we ingest, but from suppressed feelings. "As the body releases toxins physically, people start to release long-held emotions as well," he says. "Along with the physical cleansing comes an emotional catharsis."

Most visitors come to Hippocrates suffering significant health problems that require more than conventional medicine. The institute's newsletter includes many testimonials from seriously ill patients who had dire prognoses but who defied the odds. A three-week stay is recommended for maximum benefit; those with less serious conditions stay one or two weeks. The institute attracts visitors from all over. A recent Sunday orientation included a French woman recovering from breast cancer, a sixteen-year-old girl with brain cancer, a morbidly obese, middle-aged man from New York, and a Polish woman just looking to stay healthy. The sixteen-year-old girl had visited before, and reported that her doctors were astonished at her improvement.

Be forewarned: Many repeat visitors sound distinctly cultish when espousing the program. One thirty-something lawyer practically chanted affirmations to himself while ladling soup into his bowl at the buffet table. "I am going to treat myself to some warm food," he said aloud, to no one in particular. "But I don't need it all the time. I recognize it is filling an emotional need."

There's no denying that after three weeks, many visitors report a new glow to their skin and a sparkle in their eyes, saying they can't recall ever feeling so revitalized. Hippocrates documents their changes with an impressive array of before-and-after photos. "No one comes here and just gets cured," says Brian Clement. "But thousands come and heal themselves. What you're paying for is support and education on how to take care of yourself."

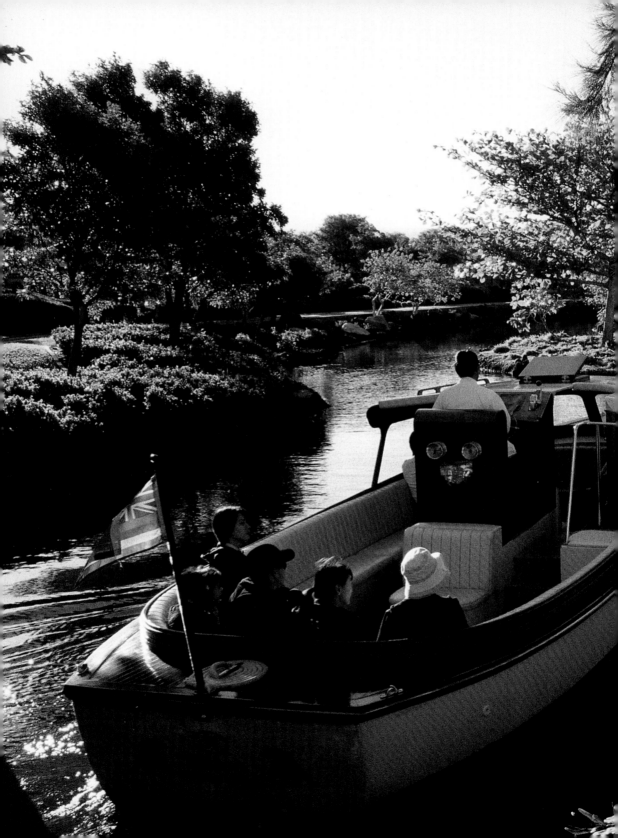

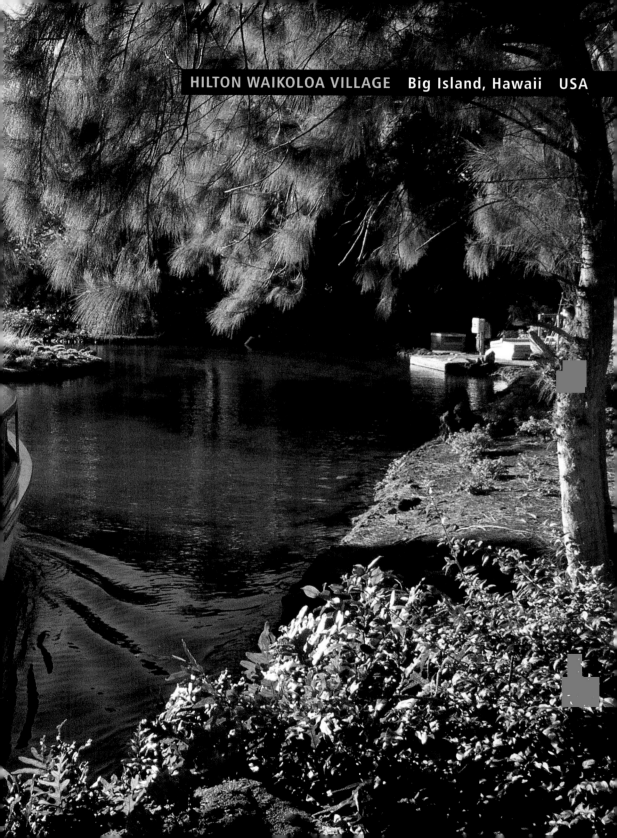

HILTON WAIKOLOA VILLAGE, WAIKOLOA, BIG ISLAND

Once upon a time, Waikoloa Village had a "living Buddha" on its Vegas-like grounds. When it first opened in 1988, the original owner, an avid art collector who bought many Buddha statues for the resort, asked a tai chi master by the name of Anahata to go about the property performing his fluid moves. Knees bent, raising his hands to the heavens and back down again, he would glide from one position to the next like a macho ballet dancer. Soon, the more curious of the guests began approaching Anahata in order to learn more, and thus began his teaching.

Today, one of those students, Kathy Mason, a lovely middle-aged woman from upstate New York with frosted hair and gold-rimmed glasses, teaches tai chi at Waikoloa. She credits the practice with helping to alleviate her symptoms of a genetic heart condition; she is the closest thing the resort now has to a living Buddha. Standing on a mound overlooking the volcanic rock at ocean's edge, she wears a black silk Chairman Mao jacket and radiates a solid inner calm. She instructs us to "feel the energy of the ocean in our heart center." A giant white Buddha statue sits behind us, a silent presence of peace.

Hilton's Waikoloa Village is where the Polynesian cliché of Hawaiian tourism meets the Eastern concept of spirituality—converging with the natural grace of a tai chi move. After class, you might sit poolside and sip a mai tai beneath the tiki torches. Guests can navigate the sprawling sixty-two acres via tram or waterway on an automatically navigated boat. Outdoor restaurants and sushi bars that jut out over the lagoons and swimming pools along the canal seem to go on forever, with their oodles of caves, cliffs, and waterfalls (one has a 175-foot slide).

Amid all of this, many guests take pleasure in Kathy's morning meditation walks and tai chi classes. Some return again and again just to study with her, and I can understand why. During my second meditation with her in the Zen garden (next to the Japanese restaurant, of course), I opened my eyes and looked down to see the koi bobbing in the pond; I became one with the fishes (in a good way). I was relaxed enough to feel like one of these orange-and-black-spotted creatures, suspended in time, floating, drifting aimlessly, at peace.

Everything here is spread out over the grounds so you don't feel overwhelmed by the trappings of ersatz tourism, however tasteful they may be (the auto-navigated boat is sleek mahogany, after all). The $7 million collection of Asian art on display throughout adds superb character and charm to a place that might otherwise look like just another splashy vacation resort. Much of the art is showcased in a three-quarter-mile museum walkway, an open-air path that runs along the ocean. Here, you're shielded from the sun, and a beautiful Big Island breeze ruffles the air as you walk past Thai carvings of bodhisattvas (enlightened beings),

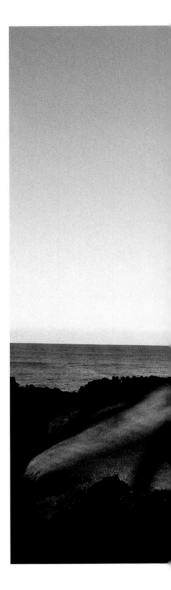

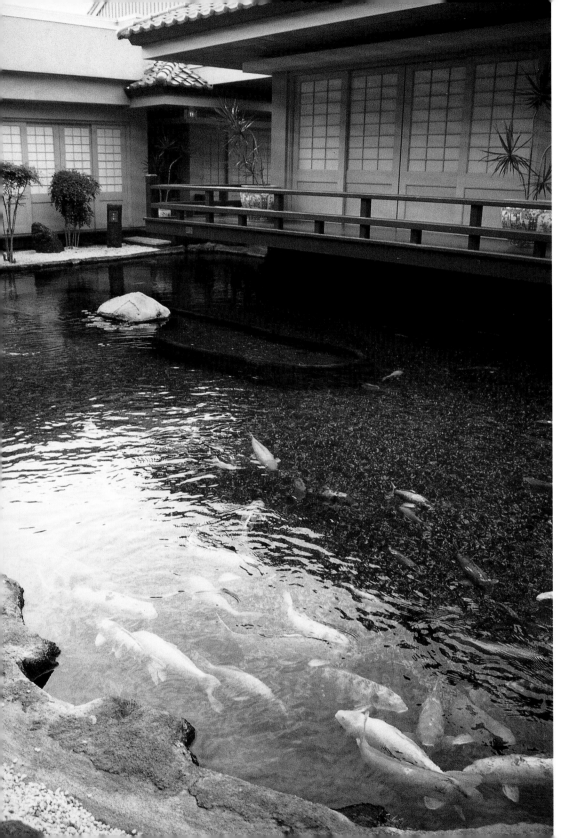

THIS SPA IS FOR YOU IF you want to explore the facets of meditation at a traditional and elegant Hawaiian resort.

THIS SPA IS NOT FOR YOU IF you desire a nice little getaway where you can tumble right into the ocean.

red lacquered Chinese wedding trays, and sculptures of fat Japanese warriors with comically mean faces. The eye is further entranced by an array of porcelain vases with gold elephant-tusk handles, carved, gilded gates from the castles of Indian rajas, and Burmese mosaics of silver and gold sequins. All this to take in on the way to the dolphin petting pool, the snorkeling lagoon, and the Kohala Sports Club and Spa.

One drawback to all of this is that though the power of the ocean is invoked everywhere, the rocky volcanic coast is unsuitable for swimming. Not to worry: For those wanting to swim, a shuttle will provide a three-minute ride to the neighboring property's beach.

While you may not be able to lie out on the sand at Waikoloa Village, you can have a massage on a cliff overlooking the sea, which is just as appealing. The sound of the ocean and that wonderful tropical breeze drifting off the waves multiplies the massage bliss factor a thousand fold. The *lomi lomi*, a traditional Hawaiian massage technique handed down through the centuries by *kihunas*, or healers, is a perfect indulgence by the sea, with its circular, rocking, and rolling movements. Breathe in, taking in that ocean energy again. Feel it in your heart center, as Kathy Mason would say. Afterwards, you can sip a mai tai and learn the hula.

PRICE $$$–$$$$

ROOMS 1,240
Elegantly appointed.

FOOD
Nine restaurants, ranging from Italian to Japanese, from Chinese to Hawaiian regional. **THE KAMUELA PROVISION CO.** has a great romantic outdoor setting practically on the beach— try the appetizer selection for two with "volcano-seared" ahi, roasted shrimp, and a lobster martini.

OUTSTANDING TREATMENTS
Lomi Lomi Massage, ocean-side; Ti-Leaf Cooling Wrap (great after too much sun); Orchid Isle Body Wrap (uses silky-oil from the ubiquitous Hawaii orchid).

ACTIVITIES
Snorkeling in the hotel's lagoon; Interacting with bottlenose dolphins on-site; Whale-Watching Cruise; Horseback Riding; Helicopter Ride over volcanoes; Golf on two 18-hole championship courses and a putting course; and eight Tennis Courts.

CLASSES
Golf-Strengthening for a better swing; Hula Lessons; Heartmath Biofeedback Session (learn relaxation through monitoring heart rate); Yoga; Tai Chi; Aqua-Aerobics; and Swiss Ball (similar to Pilates using a giant rubber ball as prop).

NEARBY ATTRACTIONS
Hawaii Volcanoes National Park (a 3-hour drive or 45-minute helicopter tour).

FOR CHILDREN
Camp Menehune offers daily and evening activities for ages 5–12.

CONFERENCE SPACE
Banquet halls seat up to 2,000.

GETTING THERE
A 30-minute drive from Kona airport; Direct flights from California and Honolulu on Aloha Airlines and Hawaii Airlines.

ADDRESS
425 Waikoloa Beach Drive Waikoloa, HI 96738

T 800-HILTONS   **F** 808-886-2900   **E** info@hiltonwaikoloavillage.com   **W** www.hiltonwaikoloavillage.com

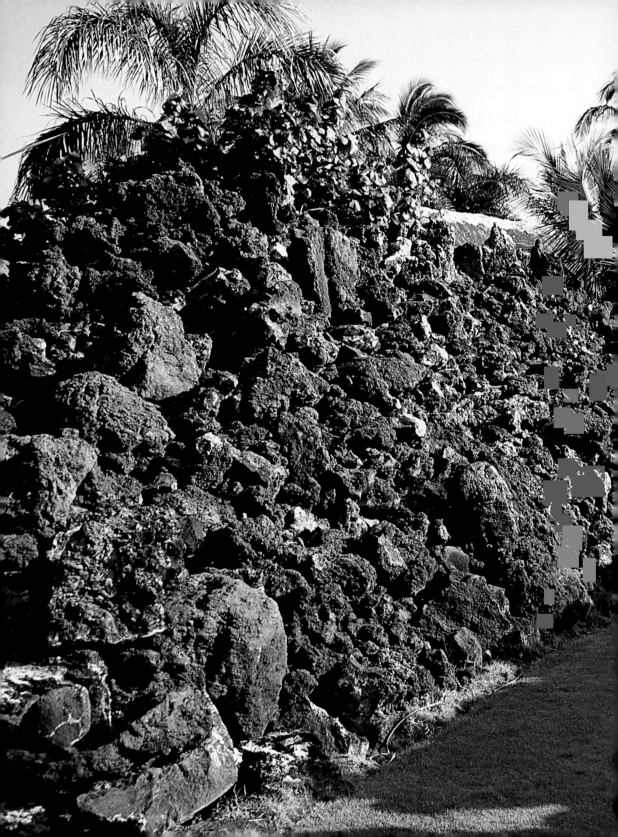

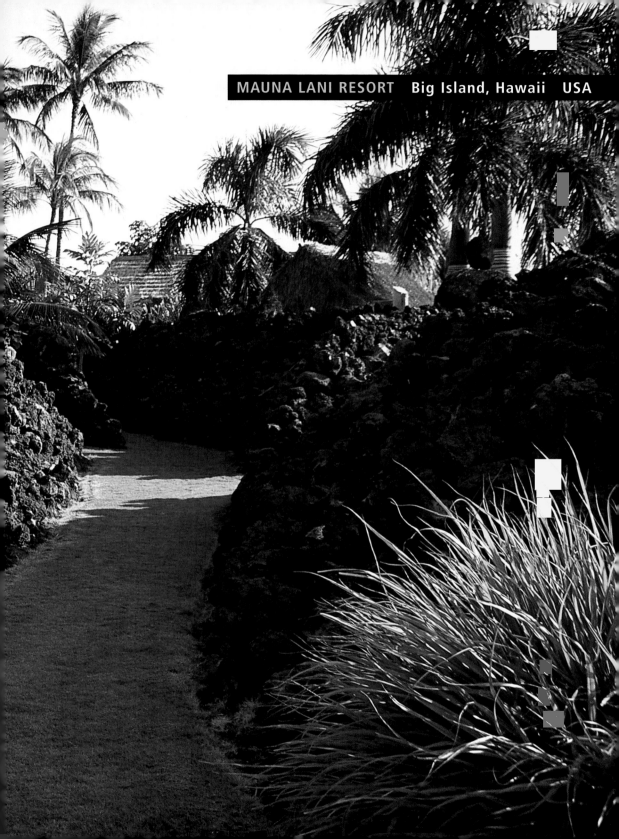

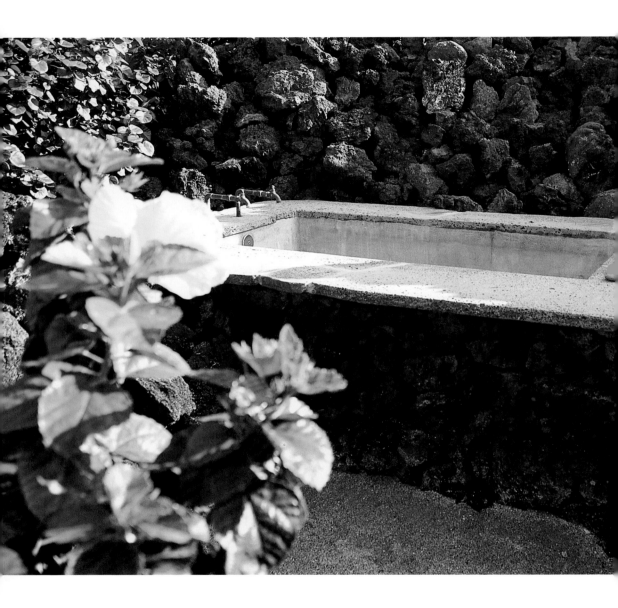

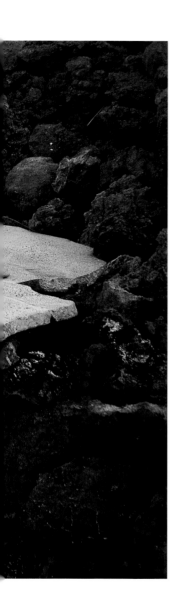

MAUNA LANI RESORT, KOHALA COAST, BIG ISLAND

The Big Island is a peaceful place that rose from a fiery, violent past—much like Hawaii itself, formed by volcanic eruptions from the seafloor. According to legend, these eruptions were the result of the goddess Pele's explosive temper; each time she went into a rage, another island was created.

It is believed she now makes her home in Kilauea, currently Hawaii's most active volcano. Three hours from Kilauea (the Big Island is as large as the state of Connecticut), the Mauna Lani Resort displays its own molten lava at the indoor-outdoor spa. Situated on land formed by a sixteenth-century lava flow, the spa is a masterpiece of natural beauty that showcases Hawaii's rich abundance of healing plants. The spa resembles the tropical jungles of Thailand or Bali. Its nine *hales*, thatched huts used as treatment rooms, feature shiny wood floors, and are surrounded inside and out with hibiscus, plumeria (used for leis), and banana trees.

Mauna Lani solves one of the more agonizing dilemmas of a spa vacation: As much as you might enjoy spending a whole afternoon at a spa, sometimes you feel like you're missing the scenery of a new place. It's hard to leave the beautiful outdoors for the cave-like womb of a spa. At Mauna Lani, you can have your spa and your scenery too. (Unless you want a wrap treatment; most of them are done indoors.)

Though longtime guests complain the new spa is too far from the hotel, most find the three-minute shuttle or five-minute walk worth it. One wanders a maze of lava stone walls set in lush green grass to the hales and outdoor showers (also made of gorgeous coal-black lava) where birds caw and the smell of jasmine (*pikake* in Hawaiian) delights the senses, and breadfruit leaves and bougainvillea peek out everywhere. Transformation is truly in the air. The staff is trained by a student of a *kihuna*, or traditional Hawaiian healer (the word translates as "keeper of the secret"). And the lava-stone walls were built by underprivileged youth of the island. "They really got into making little vignettes, flowers, bunnies, and faces with the rocks," recalls spa designer Sylvia Sepielli.

Another creative use of the lava rocks was the construction of an outdoor sauna or *berm*, a circular bench set in the garden sun. After putting on a *kikepa* (a sarong worn in lieu of a robe), you sit in the berm provided with your own personal coconut-shell of mud mixed with aloe vera and sandalwood—Canadian mud, as Hawaiian mud has too much glass in its volcanic ash. You're also left with a banana-leaf filled with fresh fruit salad, a drink, and a bucket of ice. Oh, yes—and a giant hibiscus to tuck behind your ear. As the sun beats down, you can pour some ice on the caked mud of your body. This contrast epitomizes the "fire and ice" theme with which the spa initially promoted itself, alluding to the snowy peaks of Mauna Kea and the volcano Mauna Loa, both nearby. *Mauna Lani* means "mountains reaching heaven."

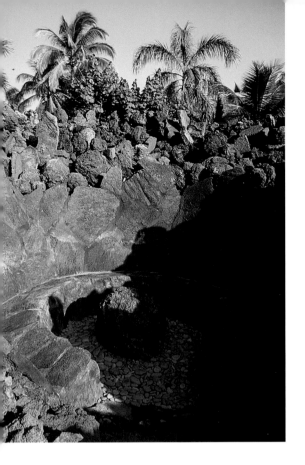

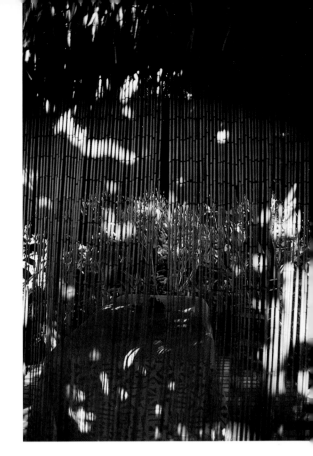

PRICE $$$–$$$$$

ROOMS 350
Elegantly appointed. Five
bungalows also available.

FOOD
Five restaurants, ranging
from very expensive
Pacific Rim to poolside
grill. All are on the
expensive side.

**OUTSTANDING
TREATMENTS**
Outdoor Lava Sauna;
Lomi Lomi Hula
(recommended for
couples—*lomi lomi* is

massage, in this case
combined with music);
Pu'olo Pa'akai (a scrub
using Hawaiian rock salt)
followed by massage using
warm stone and cool
leho (shells); Cocanilla
Experience (scrub and
wrap with coconut, sugar,
and vanilla beans); and
Plush Papaya Pineapple
Body Facial.

ACTIVITIES
Scuba Diving; Snorkeling;
Deep-Sea Fishing; Whale-
Watching Cruise; Sunset
Sails; Fish-Feeding Tours of
hotel ponds stocked with

sharks, stingrays, and
endangered *honu*
(Hawaiian green sea
turtles); two 18-hole
Golf Courses; and
ten Tennis Courts.

CLASSES
Art; Watercolor; Hula;
Lomi Lomi; Lei-Making;
Hawaiian Quilting;
Golf and Tennis Clinics;
Aqua-Aerobics;
Pilates; and Yoga.

NEARBY ATTRACTIONS
Hawaii Volcanoes National
Park (a 3-hour drive, or
45-minute helicopter tour),

Stargazing on
snow-capped Mauna Kea.

FOR CHILDREN
Camp Mauna Lani for
ages 5–12.

GETTING THERE
A 30-minute drive from
Kona airport; Direct flights
from California and
Honolulu on Aloha Airlines
and Hawaii Airlines.

ADDRESS
68-1400 Mauna Lani Drive
Kohala Coast, Hawaii
96743-9796

T 808-885-6622   **F** 808-881-7000   **E** reservations@maunalani.com   **W** www.maunalani.com

I was skeptical of playing Hawaiian dress-up and sitting outside with mud all over my body. But as birds chirped and palm trees rustled, I began to relax. "Let me know if you need more mud," the attendant told me. I looked into the coconut bowl and thought I would need very little of it. But to my surprise, I kept on slathering, almost compulsively, as I sipped ice tea and ate pineapple slices. After washing it off in the outdoor shower, I felt renewed, softer, and lighter. Then it was on to the outdoor waiting area, a meditation garden, which was a large thatched hut that had the feel of a rambling Southern porch, rocking chairs and all. The outdoor berm treatment is indeed a great way to get into the aloha spirit.

Indoors, the spa is all cozy Asian elegance, with orchids and fruit bowls everywhere. A calming *cocanilla* scrub and wrap, made from coconut pulp, vanilla beans, sugar, and oils, had me feeling like a giant cookie baking in the oven. (The coconut, alas, was fresher than what I'd had in my piña colada the night before.)

Across from the spa is a state-of-the-art fitness club offering lush tropical views, but you can also get in some exercise by walking along the paths that line historic fishponds. The ponds, created by lava hundreds of years ago, are lagoons beside the sea that hold fresh water from the surrounding mountains. They once were a plentiful food source for the Hawaiians; Hawaii's first king, Kamehameha, used this property as his country retreat—his eighteenth-century Camp David.

Mauna Lani still attracts the high and mighty, chiefly for its five private bungalows with their new, private fishponds, as well as pools and hot tubs. The two-bedroom, three-bath bungalows, costing $4,000 a night, have hosted the likes of Steven Spielberg, Kevin Costner, and other celebrities and CEOs. At that cost, one might expect a chandelier and a grand piano, yet the bungalows are understated, containing plush beige and taupe chairs and couches, as well as other furniture made from *koa*, a scarce Hawaiian tree. What one does get for the money is a twenty-four-hour butler, who will have your favorite food and music awaiting your arrival. He's been known to find grapes without skins for one guest.

Even Pele would be well-satisfied here.

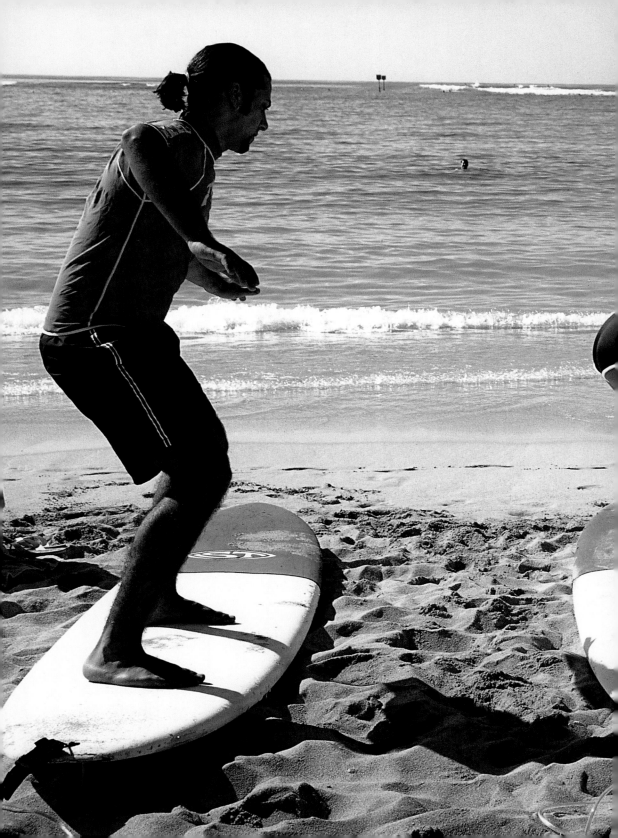

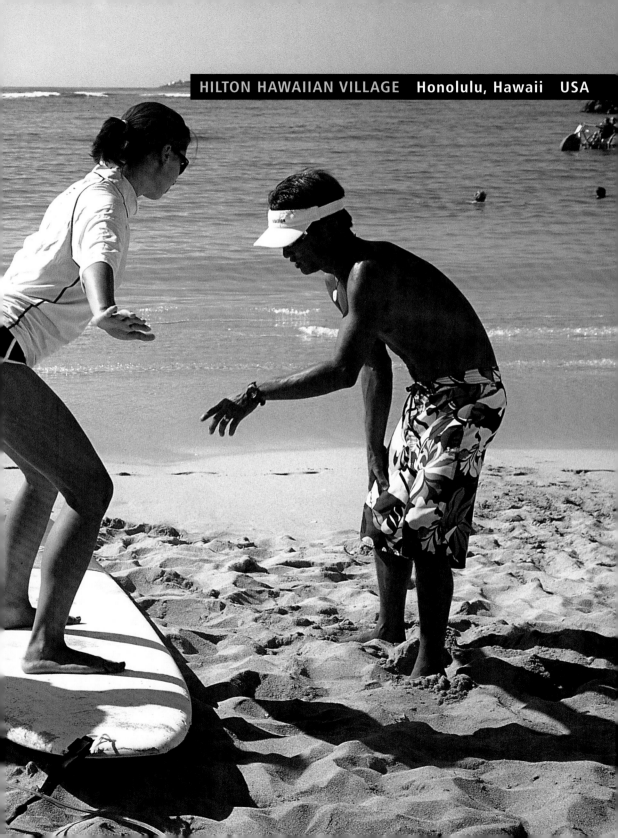

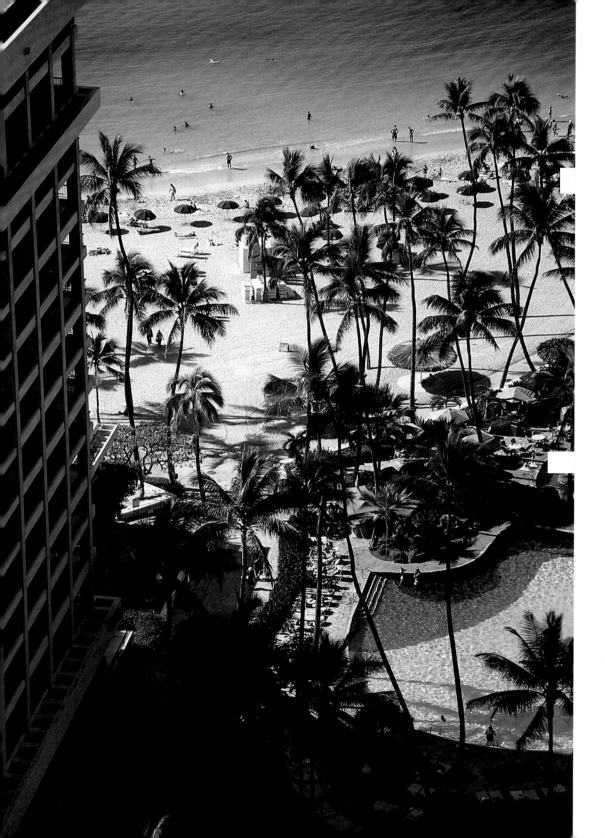

HILTON HAWAIIAN VILLAGE, HONOLULU, OAHU

Hilton calls this a village, but it's really a small city, one of the most laid-back you'll ever visit. On twenty-two acres are set six towers, each with its own lobby and a few hundred rooms. A stone path winds its way through the complex, flanked by orchids, palm trees, and lagoons populated with miniature penguins, pink flamingos, and turtles. As you stroll along, you can visit over ninety shops selling Louis Vuitton luggage, Harley-Davidson fashion accessories, and every conceivable color and print combination found on a Hawaiian shirt. There's also a village-within-a-village, the Rainbow Bazaar, a Polynesian-inspired shopping promenade.

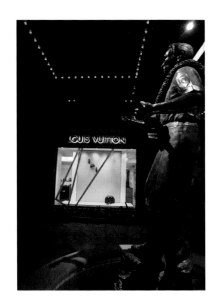

If this all sounds too much like Manhattan-meets-Hawaii, do not despair. Eventually, the stone path will lead you to Waikiki Beach, a crescent-shaped slice of smooth sand that meets the gleaming turquoise of the Pacific Ocean. Much has changed since Deborah Kerr and Burt Lancaster sealed their love on the shores of Eternity Beach. The hotels are larger and there are more of them, but Waikiki still has enough balmy charm to make you forget the crowds.

There's nothing like following a morning of shopping with a day at the beach, capped off by a Blue Hawaii cocktail. As the sun goes down, Happy Hour starts with bare-chested men darting from one tiki torch to the next, filling them with flames of fire. Friday evening, reenactments of Hawaiian royalty rituals, as well as hula and fire dancers will dazzle the kids.

Hilton Village offers a good deal more than fun and games. It can also be a place to assess your health in a pressure-free environment, thanks to Holistica, one of the resort's two spas, staffed by doctors and medical technicians. Spend the morning shopping for the perfect sarong; afterwards, head for Holistica and have a bone-density scan. Or before heading to the beach with your favorite SPF lotion, have your arteries checked for blockage. You can even have a virtual colonoscopy (less invasive than the traditional one) between yoga and surf lessons.

Holistica's biggest draw is the Electronic Beam Tomograph (EBT)—a $2 million, state-of-the-art, non-invasive scanning device used to examine calcified plaque in the heart and arteries, and used as well to detect tumors and other problems in their early stages. The EBT is also used to gauge bone density. Holistica stresses that it is not a treatment center, but a clinic with a focus on prevention and early detection. At the same time, staff proudly share stories of case histories like that of a fifty-nine-year-old man, an avid hiker who appeared healthy. Yet doctors found that 60 percent of his coronary arteries were blocked—putting him at high risk for heart disease. Fortunately, there was still time for him to reverse the damage.

Visitors to Holistica are mostly busy executives who can't make time during the work week to deal with health issues. (If you do receive unsettling news, the spa will refer

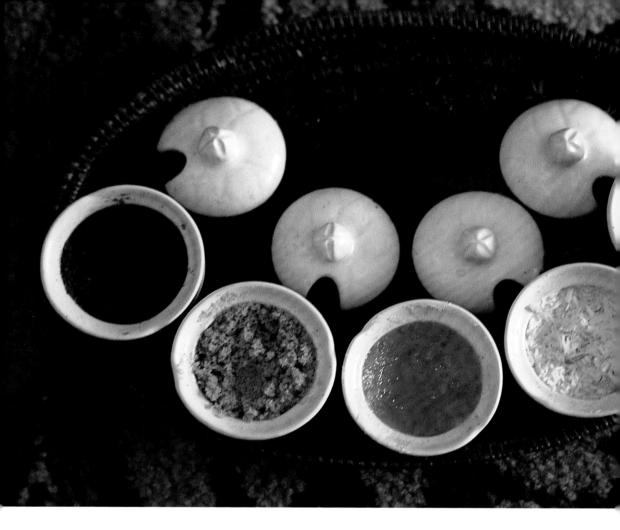

PRICE $$–$$$$

ROOMS 3,432
Mostly basic,
clean & pleasant.

FOOD
Sixteen restaurants with a
wide range: escargot
mushroom purses at the
gourmet eatery; Hawaiian
barbecue buffet; hot dogs
and curly fries by the
beach. **NIUMALU CAFE & BAR**
has tasty spa treats.

**OUTSTANDING
TREATMENTS**
Vanilla & *Pikake* Facial;
Kona Coffee Scrub; and
Chocolate Bath for Two.

ACTIVITIES
Shopping; Surfing;
Snorkeling; Kayaking;
and Sailing.

CLASSES
Wellness Lectures;
Surfing; Aqua-Aerobics;
Hula Aerobics;

Hawaiian Quilting
demonstrations;
Lei-Making.

NEARBY ATTRACTIONS
Pearl Harbor, Bishop
Museum (features history
of Waikiki).

FOR THE CHILDREN
Rainbow Express,
offering a daily supervised
activity program for
ages 5–12.

CONFERENCE FACILITIES
150,000 square feet
of space.

GETTING THERE
A 20-minute drive from
Honolulu airport.

ADDRESS
2005 Kalia Road
Honolulu, Hawaii 96815

T 808-949-4321   **F** 808-947-7898   **E** hawaii@mandaraspa.com   **W** www.hiltonhawaiianvillage.com

THIS SPA IS FOR YOU IF you love shopping, tropical breezes, and the beach.
THIS SPA IS NOT FOR YOU IF you want your own private Hawaiian hideaway.

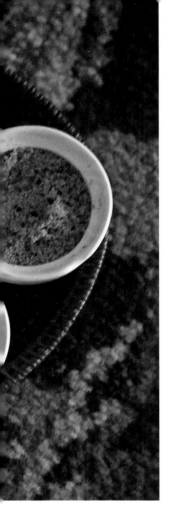

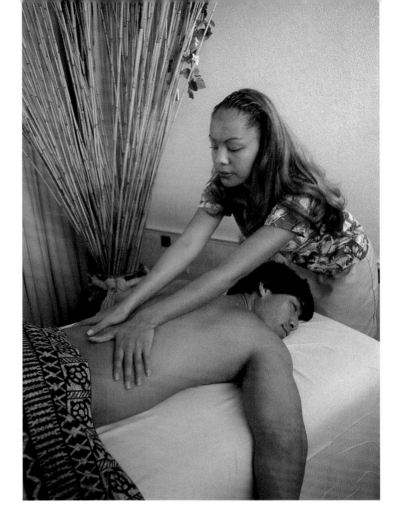

you to a doctor and provide a CD of your scan.) For some, the calming ocean breeze can help soften the blow of any unwelcome medical news.

For those who prefer a tropical holiday uninterrupted by medical scans, there's the Mandara Spa, an Asian-inspired haven offering Balinese and Hawaiian massage, vanilla facials, and jasmine-flower baths. During my vanilla facial, Larissa, my Russian aesthetician, held her very sensitive hands over my forehead and said, "Something is bothering you. I can feel you thinking."

She was right. My mind was busy, mulling over everything—from the money I had spent shopping that afternoon (when you find a bathing suit that looks good, you have to buy it!) to whether or not to have the pineapple chicken for dinner at the Hawaiian buffet. Not even Holistica's EBT scanner is that sensitive.

I confessed my worries to Larissa, who leaned over and whispered softly in my ear: "Forget it. Let it go."

So I did.

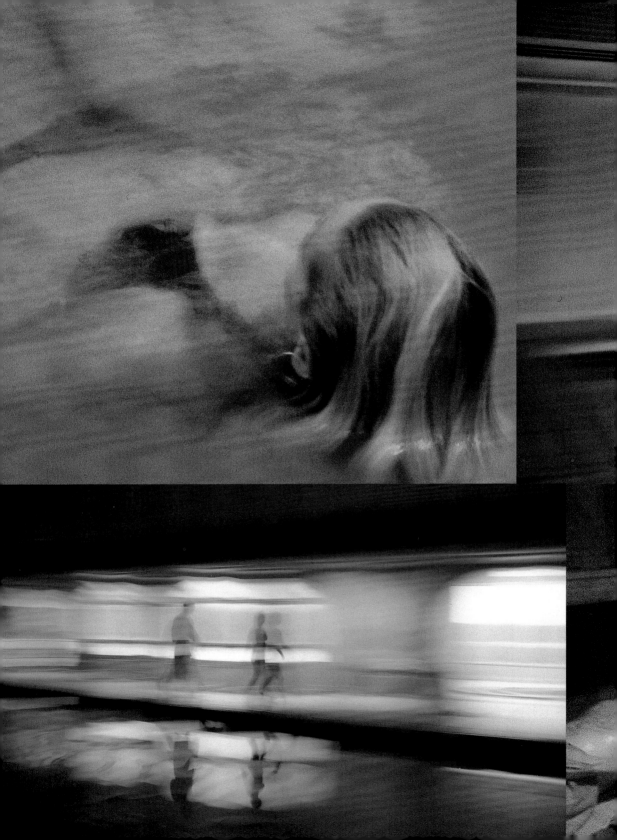

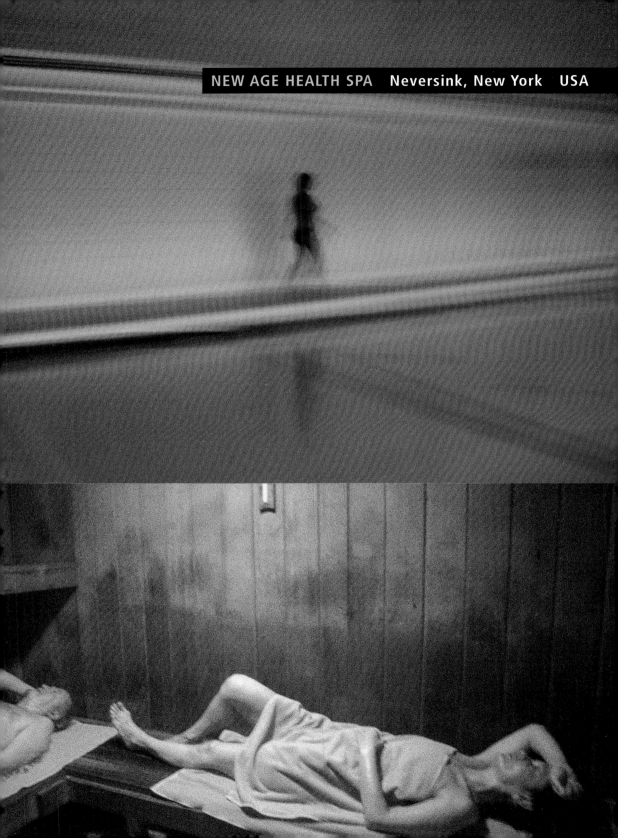

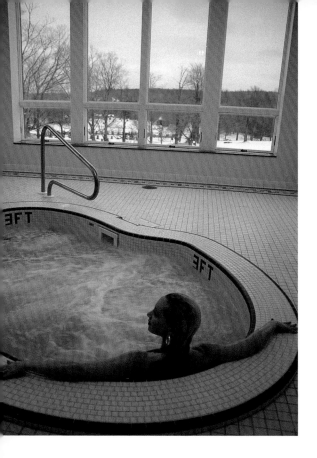

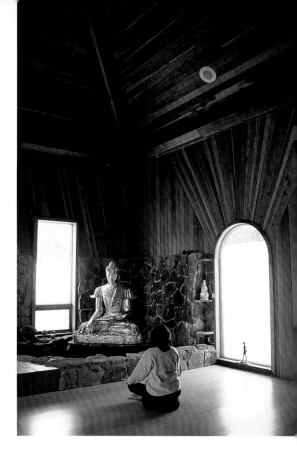

PRICE $$

ROOMS 37
Accommodates 72, with doubles and triples. Basic, clean & pleasant.

FOOD
Main dining room offers fresh produce from organic garden on-site. A salad buffet with a choice of soups is available for lunch and dinner.

A typical entrée might include involtini (pasta pinwheels) with roasted tomato sauce and spinach, and chicken in ginger-coconut sauce.

OUTSTANDING TREATMENTS
Maple Sugar Body Polish.

CLASSES
Cabaret Dancing; Pranayama; Ai-Chi (water

exercise and relaxation class); Tai Chi; Chi Kung; Pilates; and Yoga. Nightly lectures are offered on nutrition, anti-aging, and the sorts of subjects you might expect at a New Age spa, like "Life Regression" and "Psychic Phenomena."

ACTIVITIES
Bird-Watching; Climbing the Alpine Tower

(a jungle-gym-type contraption for climbing—offered in summer only); Greenhouse Tour; Hiking; Horseback Riding (off-site, one hour away).

GETTING THERE
A 2 1/2-hour drive from New York City.

ADDRESS
Route 55
Neversink, NY 12765

T 800-682-4348   **F** 845-985-2467   **E** office@newagehealthspa.com   **W** www.newagehealthspa.com

THIS SPA IS FOR YOU IF you seek a reasonably priced place for quiet reflection, as well as a good dose of health and fitness—either by yourself or with friends.

THIS SPA IS NOT FOR YOU IF you desire four-star service or access to many outside activities.

NEW AGE HEALTH SPA, NEVERSINK

During my first visit to New Age, I made the acquaintance of an Italian journalist who had visited many spas all over the world. What brought her to this quiet, unassuming spa in upstate New York? "This one is pure," she said.

Pure? No, it wasn't poor English on her part. Many spa-goers consider no-frills accommodations and juice fasts to be pure. New Age started in 1976 as one of the first American retreats where one could learn yoga and meditation, and cleanse the colon with vegetable juices.

Today, New Age has new owners and has undergone several renovations, but it remains true to its roots. Juice fasts are optional, and delicious, healthy meals from the organic gardens are now offered, but the spa retains the atmosphere of a rustic retreat. Most of the accommodations are basic, comfortable hotel rooms with no phones or TVs. With the exception of a giant gold Buddha in the newly renovated yoga studio, there's not much in the way of decorative detail.

Yet stroll about the storybook setting of this 280-acre Catskill preserve—particularly in winter, when snow covers the ground and wind chimes echo in the crisp air like whispering church bells—and you'll find many of nature's decorative touches. A breeze gusts and giant pines shake the powdery snow from their branches. True, the white vinyl lodgings clustered in a small corner of the landscape are not the most scenic, but they do not distract from the natural beauty of the place.

In winter, snowshoeing can prove to be a spiritual experience as well as a great aerobic workout. The opaque purple glow of the setting sun, with glints of light that break through miles of grand pines, provides nature's own stained-glass window. Walking atop the snow with an endless vista before you is the perfect way to become one with nature, almost like melting into it. Afterwards, Anne Walsemann's tai chi class offers a graceful counterpoint to the trudging, stomping movements of snowshoeing. As you bring your hands in front of your heart and lift one leg before flowing sideways, you can gaze out of the studio window at acres of snow-covered meadows.

This pristine nature can inspire a diet to match, and the spa is fairly strict about what is consumed. A sign at the entrance instructs visitors to leave all drugs, candy, and cigarettes in a nearby receptacle. Alcohol is prohibited, but juices, such as beet, fennel, and a celery mix, are prepared to resemble Caribbean cocktails.

All of this purity inspired me to try my first colonic. Linda Troeller, the photographer for this book, swears colonics have cured her of all sorts of ills. Yet like most who have never tried one, I thought the very idea of a colonic bizarre. But a spa journeyer must be open to all things.

The procedure itself was painless, except for some mild abdominal cramps. Sue Martin, a trained nurse who works in a cardiologist's office during the week, chatted with me about her family's Christmas festivities as she cleaned my innards. The objective is to cleanse the digestive system of toxic buildup. Proponents of the treatment claim detritus can cling to intestinal walls for decades. (One therapist told of a client who was purged of a plastic Barbie shoe). "I undergo them myself," said Sue, "and afterwards, I feel so much better. I swear I can even *see* better."

I felt the same way: lighter and clearer. Later, however, I found Linda, fresh from her procedure, looking utterly miserable and curled in the fetal position on a waiting-room couch. I was later told that sometimes the toxins from the intestines escape into the bloodstream, where the body takes longer to eliminate them.

I felt so good when I returned home that I thought nothing of indulging in two glasses of wine, some cheese, and a little chocolate. The next morning I felt hung over, and curled up on the couch like Linda had. How I yearned again for the pure, pristine regimen of New Age.

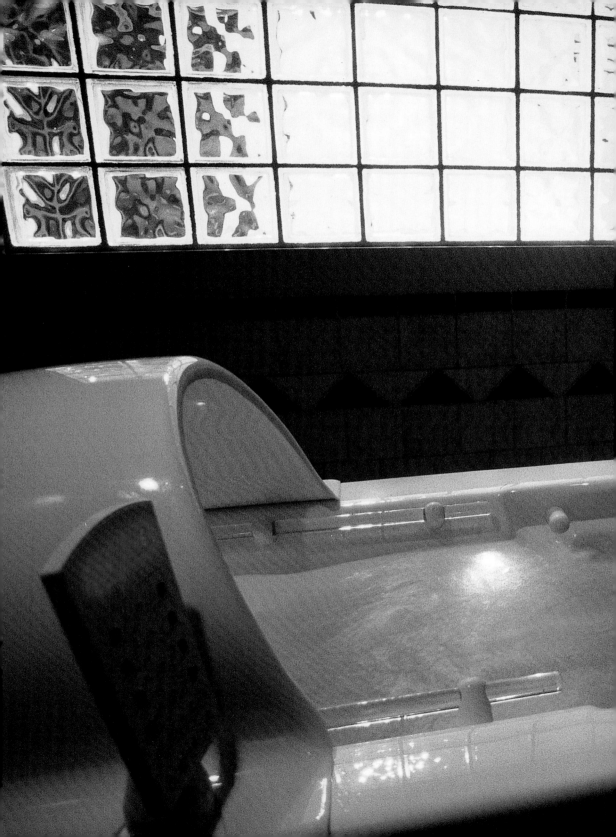

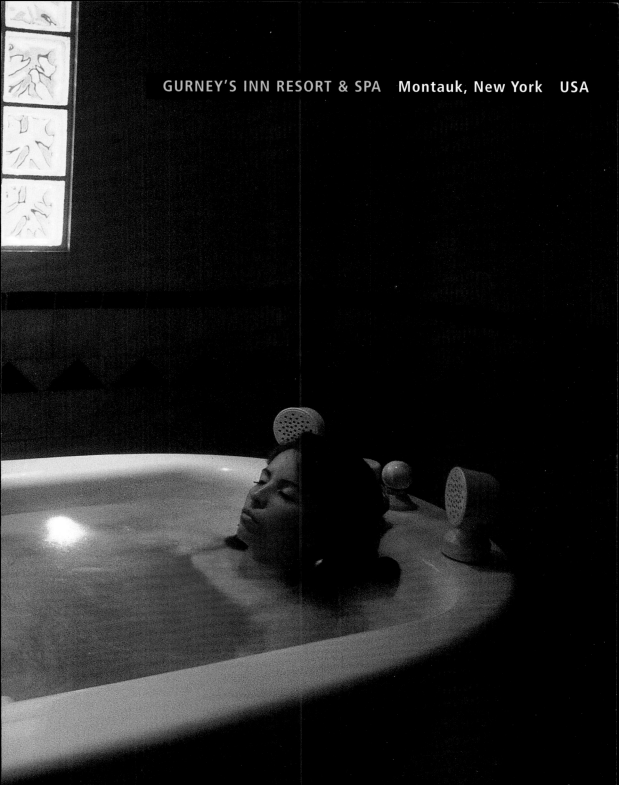

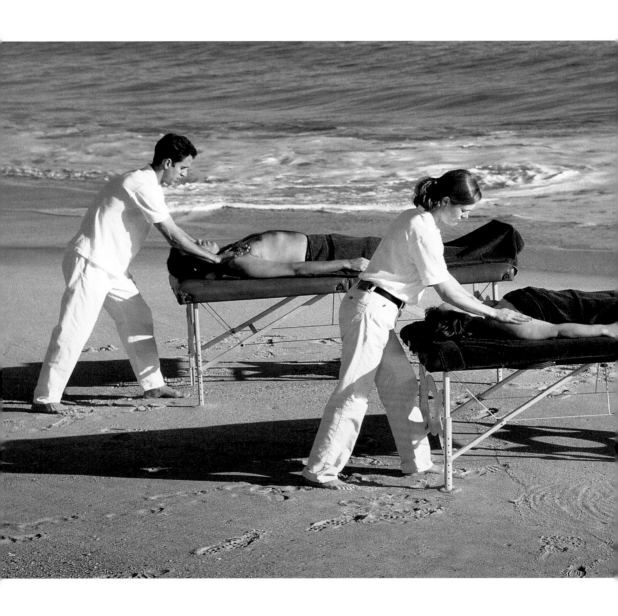

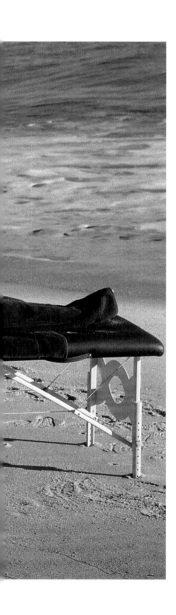

GURNEY'S INN RESORT & SPA, MONTAUK

Seaweed gel, micronized to seep into the skin, coats your body like heavy cream, making you feel like a glazed mermaid. The smell of algae, a tad unpleasant, competes with that of lavender—the ubiquitous spa scent. The gel is full of minerals thought to detoxify and purify the skin—"sea nutrients," your hostess says proudly.

Gurney's, the only thalassotherapy spa in the United States, is perched high on a cliff above the sea, and thus perfectly situated to offer this particular therapy, which uses seawater and marine plants in a range of treatments. The Olympic-size pool draws fresh ocean water from an underground reserve, and thousands of people come each year to soak up such nutrients as magnesium, calcium, and potassium. If you prefer, you can soak in the seawater in your own private bath, and alter the room to your mood. Instead of the dark green of the ocean, turn the water pink, blue, or bright green in a nod to color therapy. "Color really affects the mood," says Ingrid Lemme, Gurney's public-relations director. "Many guests don't want to feel they're bathing in the ocean."

Though American doctors are known to be skeptical, many European physicians swear by thalassotherapy for the treatment and prevention of such afflictions as osteoporosis and hypertension. Gurney's staffs a full-time nurse at the pool who conducts physical-therapy sessions for local guests. "Many local doctors will refer patients here," says spa nurse Susan Yonkers. "Exercise in heated water allows for an easier and more intense workout and can increase circulation and stimulate the kidneys. We try to get the word out so that more doctors in the U.S. will be open to thalassotherapy's benefits."

Gurney's also attracts celebrities from the glamorous Hamptons, some twenty minutes west. Many stop by just for the day, perhaps while visiting Steven Spielberg and Barbra Streisand, who have homes nearby.

They come for the top-notch spa services as well as the romantic isolation of Gurney's Montauk beach. Traditionally, thalassotherapy includes breathing the sea air, and Montauk's beaches are the perfect place to do so. Teddy Roosevelt and 29,000 other veterans came here to recuperate after the Spanish-American War.

Although it's right next door, Montauk, at the eastern tip of Long Island, is the "un-Hamptons." You won't find tiny designer shops and overpriced ice cream—just patches of long sea-grass dotting the bluffs and gulls hovering in the sky overhead. The town is still a fishing village, offering a pizza parlor, a drug store, and a few boxy motels.

For those who do not relish being smothered in seaweed-gel, algae-mud, or any other kind of lotion from the sea, the beach at Gurney's is one of the finest in the Northeast. Carved cliffs stand guard over powdery dunes, and waves swipe at the sand like lion's paws, unleashing a quiet roar. Just lie back, inhale, and let the sea air do the rest.

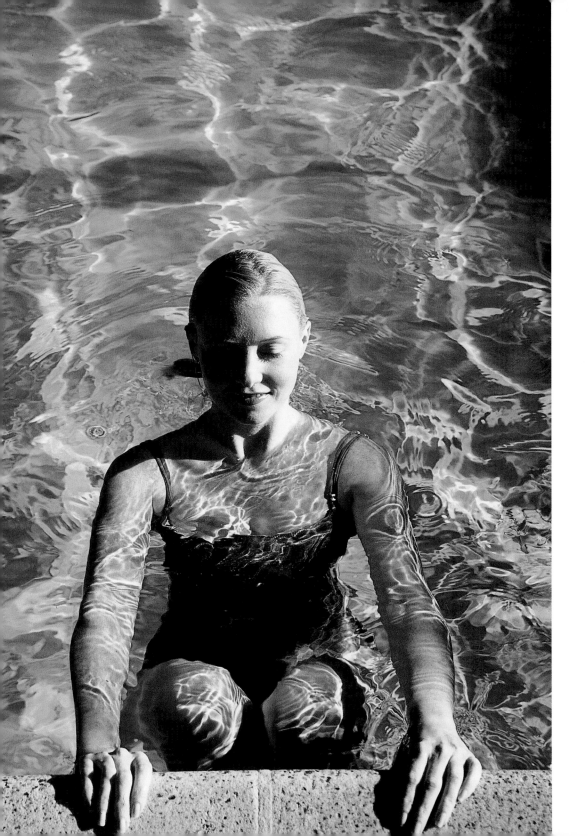

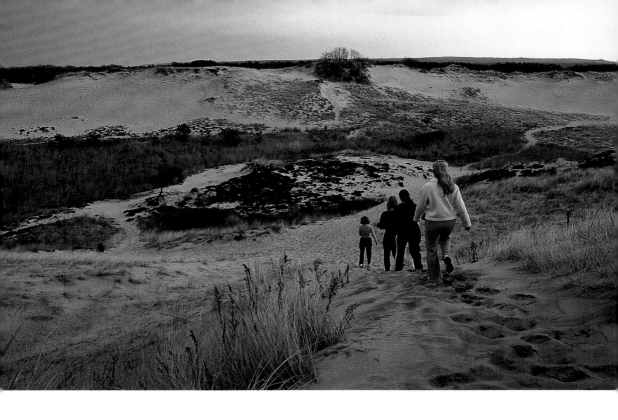

PRICE $$$

ROOMS 109
Basic, clean & pleasant.
Many offer spectacular
ocean views.

FOOD
Seafood is the specialty in
the main dining room
(lobster is a favorite).
Spa cuisine is available.

**OUTSTANDING
TREATMENTS**
Thalasso Hydro-Therapy
Massage; Seaweed Wrap;
and Ocean Radiance
Facial.

ACTIVITIES
Biking; Lighthouse Walk
(over rocks); 18-hole public
Golf Course; and
Horseback Riding nearby.

CLASSES
Aqua-Aerobics;
Tai Chi; and Yoga.

NEARBY ATTRACTIONS
Montauk Lighthouse
(built in 1797 by order of
George Washington);
the Hamptons.

CONFERENCE SPACE
Six event rooms for up to
350 guests.

GETTING THERE
A 2 1/2 to 3-hour drive
from New York City
(weekend traffic often
causes delays).

ADDRESS
290 Old Montauk Highway
Montauk, NY 11954

T 800-8-GURNEY   **F** 631-668-3576   **E** info@gurneys-inn.com   **W** www.gurneys-inn.com

THIS SPA IS FOR YOU IF you love the ocean and you want a quick getaway from New York City.

THIS SPA IS NOT FOR YOU IF you want some real sightseeing, and beachcombing and celebrity-spotting is not enough.

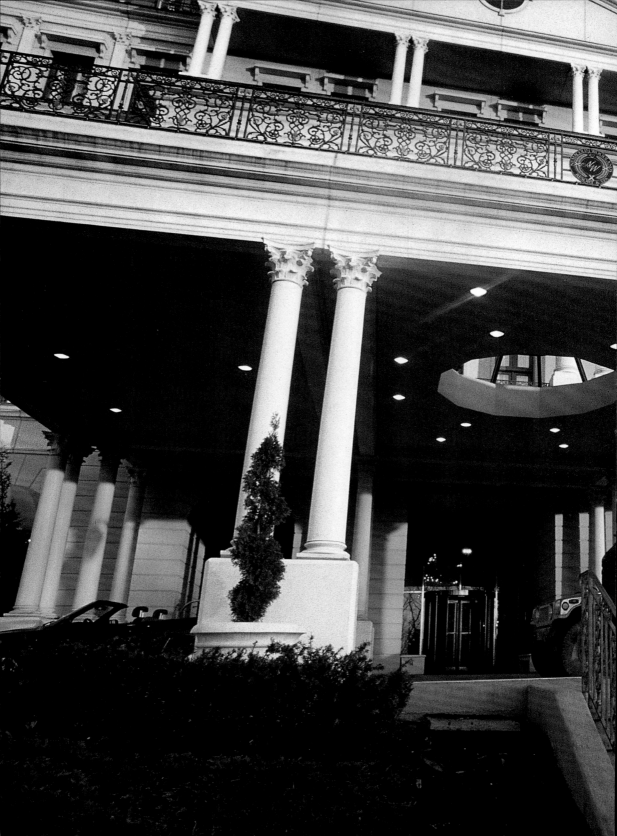

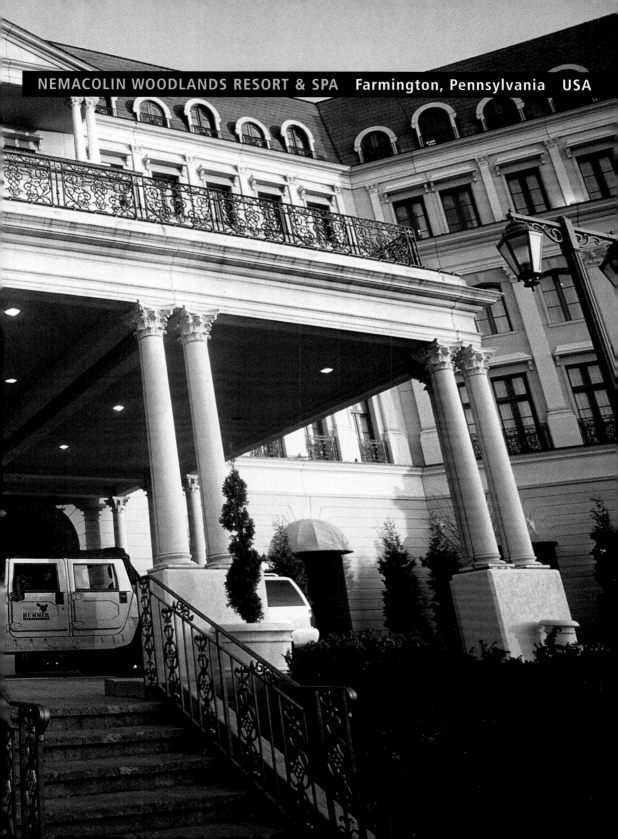

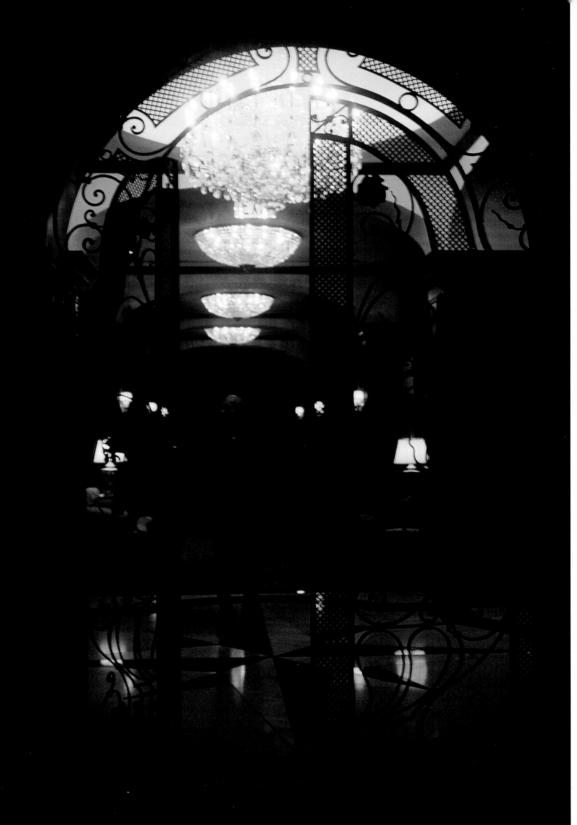

NEMACOLIN WOODLANDS RESORT & SPA, FARMINGTON

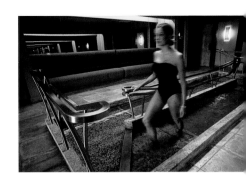

A French classical château modeled after Versailles. An English lodge with animal heads over the fireplace. An Asian retreat so meticulously designed that the door handles are carved to correspond with acupressure points on the hand. Which one is Nemacolin? All of the above—and with no clashing or confusion. On top of that, there is a children's wing with a neon jukebox, a bowling alley, and the world's largest, freestanding, cylindrical saltwater aquarium.

This bastion of variety, opulence, and sophistication lies in the middle of the Laurel Mountains just outside of Pittsburgh, of all places. The various worlds that make up Nemacolin are set in 1,700 acres of rolling green hills. Each different domain has its own turf, but a change of surroundings is as quick as a walk down a hallway, or, if you're particularly ambitious, a three-mile hike through the woods. I spent hours enjoying the difference between all the buildings, as if I were in some kind of adult Disneyland. The main building has the atmosphere of a Ritz-Carlton with dark wood furniture, marble floors, and oil paintings. But walk through the sunny, chandeliered hallways into the Tudor-style lodge and you are met by hunting trophies, leather chairs, and a roaring fire. Across the way is a little cedar bridge that spans a reflecting pond surrounded by Irish moss and Norwegian pines, a storybook moat that leads to the feng shui paradise of the spa building.

Nemacolin is that rare spa resort that manages to be all things to all people—men, women, married, single, young, and old. Its golf courses are consistently rated the best in the country. It has beautiful horseback riding trails, cross-country and downhill skiing, snowboarding, fly-fishing, and a full-service shooting range. One unique adventure: For $275, you can play Indiana Jones, learning to drive an H2 Hummer for two hours through rugged terrain. During the winter holidays, kids can participate in a "Magical Land of Snow" program, building snowmen and snow castles.

A walk over the cedar bridge will bring you to the almost-sacred spa, part Buddhist temple and part luxury palace. A waterfall running down a three-story slab of copper greets you as you walk through the giant bronze doors. Renowned spa designer Clodagh says her intent was to have "water on every floor, moving in every direction," as "clear, running water symbolizes prosperity," according to feng shui. As with most Asian spas, the four elements of air, earth, fire, and water are prevalent...but mostly, there is water.

Water is the main feature of the treatments as well. Try a Kneipp treatment (alternating hot and cold water, said to stimulate the immune system), by strolling the Water Path: As you walk along this shallow built-in pool, stones massage and knead your feet and the water alternates in temperature. A subtle light show plays along with you too, with different designs and shapes beamed onto the stone floor and plaster walls, lending softness to these "earth" elements.

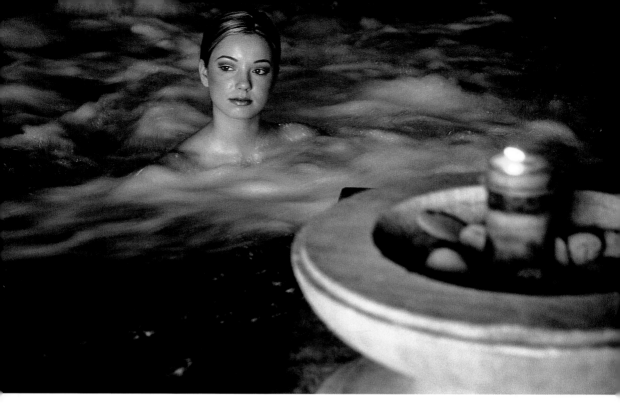

PRICE $$$

ROOMS 275
Sumptuous and
luxurious or elegantly
appointed. One- and
two-bedroom town houses
with kitchen are excellent
for families.

FOOD
Ten restaurants. French
gourmet; creative spa
food at **SEASONS**;
a cafeteria-style
buffet at the **HUNGRY
MOOSE CAFÉ**. High tea is
also served.

**OUTSTANDING
TREATMENTS**
The Water Path;
Shirodara (Indian ayurvedic
treatment in which warm
oil is poured on the
forehead); and a soak in
the Roman Bath.

ACTIVITIES
36 holes of Golf on two
PGA-rated championship
courses; Golf Academy
with lessons and clinics;
Shooting Range;
Hummer Driving Lessons;
Horseback Riding;
Skiing; Hiking; Biking;
Fishing; and Canoeing.

Whitewater Rafting and
Kayaking nearby.

CLASSES
Step Aerobics; Physio Ball;
Cardio Kick; Aqua-
Aerobics; and Yoga.

NEARBY ATTRACTIONS
Frank Lloyd Wright's
Fallingwater; Fort Necessity
(where young George
Washington was defeated
by the French in 1754).

FOR CHILDREN
The Kidz Club (ages 4–12)
offers plenty to keep
children busy and

entertained year-round,
with a ropes obstacle-
course, scavenger hunts,
hiking, biking, and an
arcade.

CONFERENCE SPACE
26,000 square feet of
meeting and banquet
space.

GETTING THERE
An hour's drive from the
Pittsburgh airport.

ADDRESS
1001 LaFayette Drive
Farmington, PA
15437-9901

T 800-422-2736   **F** 724-329-6153   **E** colon@nwlr.com   **W** www.nemacolin.com

THIS SPA IS FOR YOU IF you crave luxury, variety, and golf.
THIS SPA IS NOT FOR YOU IF you want rugged hiking with staggering views.

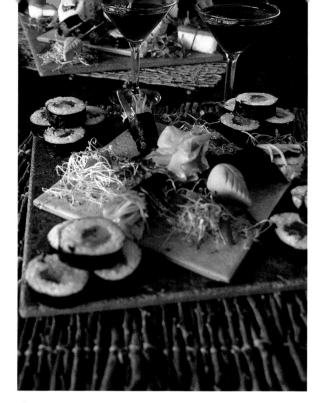

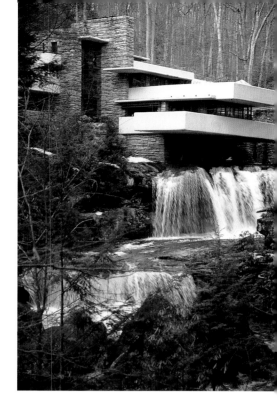

The water theme continues in the corridor leading to the spa restaurant, Seasons. A lineup of video screens with images of Frank Lloyd Wright's Fallingwater (the Kaufmann house, located nearby) are built into a wall over a pebble-strewn creek; sounds of trickling water wash over you. If you aren't feeling fluidly relaxed by now, you will be by the time you sit down in the restaurant, a work of art in itself. A giant mobile of shiny aluminum plates hangs from the ceiling, rotating at a slow, graceful pace. It was designed so that this cavernous space would feel less empty when there are fewer diners—it creates the illusion of movement throughout the room.

Seasons boasts some of the most innovative spa food in the country, with offerings like breast of pheasant marinated in pomegranate molasses; wok-seared salmon cooked in an iron Dutch oven, simmered in coconut curry broth; and spiced ahi tuna on a bed of Israeli couscous and fruit salsa. Desserts, like the crispy chocolate hazelnut napoleon, are a spectacular demonstration of just how far spa food has come from the days of fruit cups.

In keeping with its eclectic motif, the resort offers much more than spa fare. Indeed, Nemacolin has ten restaurants offering a variety of options, including gourmet French, steak and seafood, a tearoom, and a pizza parlor. If there's nothing here to please you, you can't be pleased.

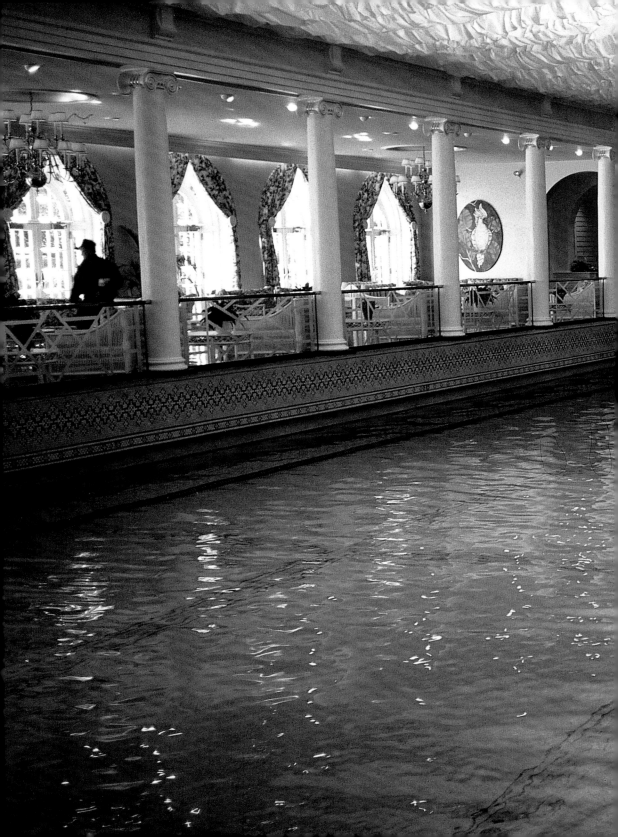

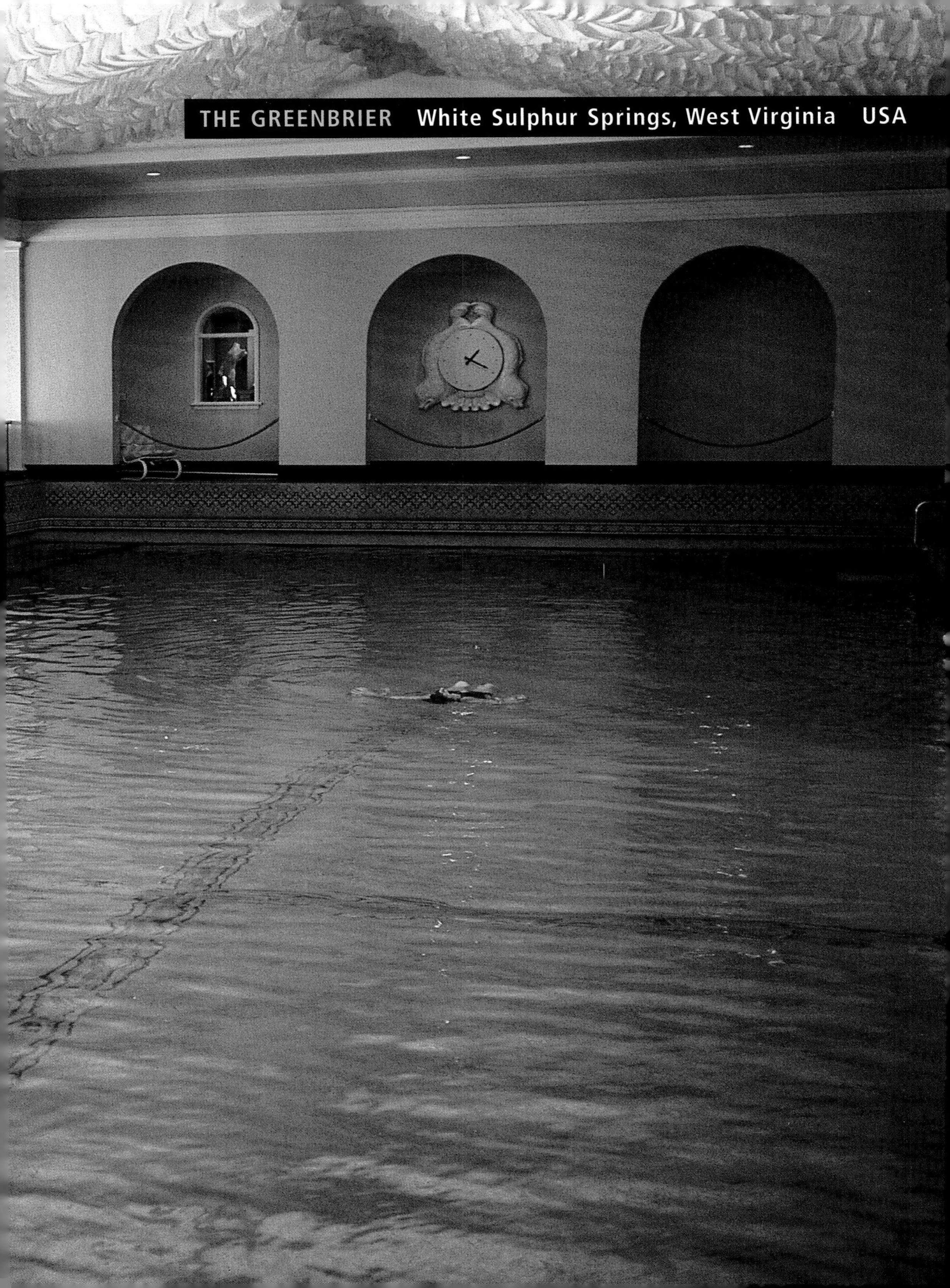

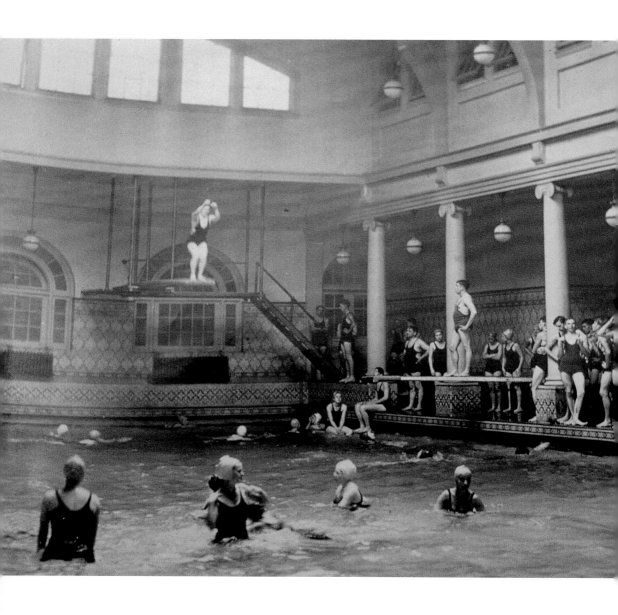

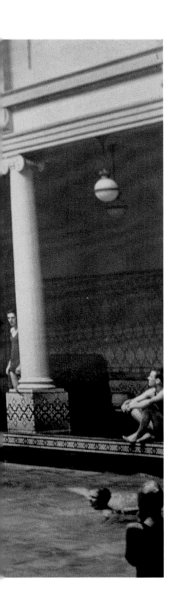

THE GREENBRIER, WHITE SULPHUR SPRINGS

From the outside, The Greenbrier resembles the White House—and in fact, it was called "the Old White Hotel" at the turn of the century, when it was the epitome of antebellum elegance. Over the years it has hosted no fewer than twelve presidents. Inside, it looks a bit like Scarlett O'Hara's beloved Tara, only more colorful. Indeed, upon entering, one is overwhelmed by colors and patterns of every description.

The Greenbrier is one-of-a-kind. Few decorators would assemble such a wide variety of fabrics in the same football field, let alone in the same lobby—which, incidentally, is nearly as large as a football field. Lemon yellow and lime green wallpaper patterned with roses and lilacs is the backdrop for a grand wrought-iron *Gone-With-the-Wind* staircase—surrounded by acres of ruby red carpeting. The unique interiors were originally decorated by designer Dorothy Draper. Her trademark floral wallpaper and vigorous palate at times give one the sensation of being inside a giant pillowcase. Wicker couches with floral-patterned cushions are set across from red leather sofas and striped chairs. Crystal chandeliers and original paintings of dukes and duchesses (by such storied American artists as Gilbert Stuart, John Singleton Copley, and John Trumbull) adorn the interior of the white-columned hotel.

The Greenbrier may be the only place where you'll ever see a sign that reads "This way to spa and bowling alley" and have it make perfect sense. Once inside the spa, the discordant color scheme becomes more subdued, but remains characteristically bright and cheery. The staff is exceptionally friendly and helpful at all times, exuding Southern hospitality and charm. For nearly two centuries, people have flocked to The Greenbrier's mineral springs. If you can stand the smell of sulfur, it's worth a try. Sulfur is pungent at first, but after a ten-minute soak most bathers become so blissfully relaxed they ignore the smell; filtered mineral water without sulfur is also available for bathing. Next, it's on to a steam or sauna (an attendant will provide a white cloth filled with ice to hold against your face); this is followed by a Swiss shower—water sprayed from every direction—and a Scotch spray—an attendant squirts a high-pressure hose at your hips, thighs, and butt (ouch, but presumably good for circulation). These treatments are capped off with an aromatherapy massage using lavender, chamomile, and ylang-ylang.

One can also drink the water in the relaxation room, from either of two spigots: one with sulfur, and one without. The spa recommends drinking only one cup or less at first, as the stuff can act as a "purgative agent."

Filtered springwater is available throughout the hotel and is served in the main dining room, which also offers some of the best food in the country. Emerald- and diamond-hued crystal chandeliers crown this sprawling room, which accommodates almost 1,100 diners. The men,

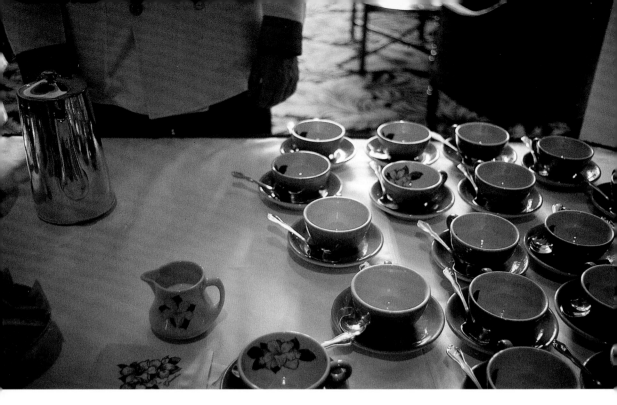

PRICE $$$$$

ROOMS 739
Including 33 suites and
96 guest houses. Elegantly
appointed.

FOOD
The main dining room
requires formal attire for
dinner and serves some of
the best food in the
country, including spa
cuisine. There is a smaller
gourmet eatery and a
separate casual restaurant
at the golf club serving
dinner. Two casual cafes
offer lunch; one is near
the swimming pool and
offers spa food; the other,
DRAPER'S, offers a selection
of yummy, rich Southern

food and desserts.
The chef will also cook
any result of your hunting,
be it pheasant, duck, or
other catch.

**OUTSTANDING
TREATMENTS**
The Greenbrier (includes
a soak in mineral springs,
sauna, Swiss shower,
Scotch spray, and
aromatherapy massage);
Haven of Peace Body
Booster (a body polish of
olive pits that leaves the
skin soft for days, and
aromatherapy massage);
Kate's Walnut Scrub
(another soft skin scrub,
this one made of crushed
walnut shells that smells
like Christmas cookies).

ACTIVITIES
Land Rover Driving Lessons;
Falconry; Clay-Pigeon
Shooting; Golf; Tennis
(five covered courts and
fifteen all-weather outdoor
courts); Horseback Riding;
Fishing; Hiking; Bowling;
Shopping at arts and crafts
stores on site; Touring
the Cold War bunker.

CLASSES
Aqua-Aerobics;
Pilates; and Yoga.

NEARBY ATTRACTIONS
Civil War historical sites in
Lewisburg; Coal-mining
museum in Beckley.

FOR CHILDREN
Supervised activities for
children 3–12.

CONFERENCE SPACE
35 meeting rooms.

GETTING THERE
The closest airport
(a 5-minute drive) is in
Lewisburg, West Virginia.
Van service to The
Greenbrier is available.
The Roanoke, VA airport is
about a 90-minute drive.
Washington, D.C. is about
a 5-hour drive.

ADDRESS
300 West Main Street
White Sulphur Springs,
WV 24986

T 304-536-1110   **F** 304-536-7854   **E** the_greenbrier@greenbrier.com   **W** www.greenbrier.com

THIS SPA IS FOR YOU IF you love luxury, mineral springs, golf, and tennis.
THIS SPA IS NOT FOR YOU IF you hate getting dressed up for dinner.

all in their required jackets, and the women, in their Sunday best, dine on impeccable food that virtually bursts with medleys of rich (read: fatty) ingredients. There is also a spa menu with choices that are quite good—baked eggplant-cannelloni stuffed with goat cheese and spinach, poached salmon, jumbo shrimp, and seafood sausage, for example—yet the less-disciplined will be tempted to sample the coq au vin with foie gras croutons, or the herb-crusted sea bass that soaks in a buttery side dish of creamed cabbage with bits of applewood-smoked bacon. For dessert, toasted-coconut pound cake with ice cream and chocolate will be a new experience for many. Or you can always stay with the familiar, such as The Greenbrier's own bread pudding, which is ecstatically flavorful.

This cloistered world of Southern luxury is set above a more-cloistered world of a different kind. In the late 1950s, President Eisenhower decided that The Greenbrier would be an ideal site to conceal a nuclear-fallout bunker for the U.S. Congress. The government camouflaged the construction by simultaneously building an additional wing. For over thirty years, this monument to Cold War terror was maintained in secrecy. In the event of a nuclear attack, the plan was for the entire U.S. Congress to decamp to this bunker, where they might survive for up to two months. When an investigative reporter revealed the location of the site in 1994 (perhaps aided by members of Congress who considered it a waste of money) the operation was shut down. A tour of the bunker is not to be missed as it offers an extraordinary trip back to the Cold War days.

Indeed, The Greenbrier is rich with history. Well before the Civil War, the lush beauty of the Allegheny Mountains and the cool air of their valleys made it a logical summer gathering place for elite Southern families. Many a belle came here as part of her "coming out," hoping to meet the beau of her dreams. The Old White Hotel was used as an infirmary during the Civil War, at first by the Confederacy, and later by Union troops. It reverted to a hospital during World War II, when the Olympic-size pool was used for physical therapy. Recovering soldiers were encouraged to take advantage of the resort's recreational facilities and some joked "golf was a mandatory formation." Today, a separate medical clinic is available to guests who can coordinate medical checkups with spa activities.

The Greenbrier became a hotel once again after the end of the war, and Draper was hired to expunge anything reminiscent of a hospital. Hence the over-the-top proliferation of bright colors and patterns. Despite the decor, the resort is as elegant as ever, at times verging on stuffy. Guests are requested to use the lower lobby when dressed for golf, tennis, riding, and other outdoor activities. Even on the indoor tennis courts, T-shirts are prohibited. But a hotel and spa that does everything right can be forgiven its peccadilloes.

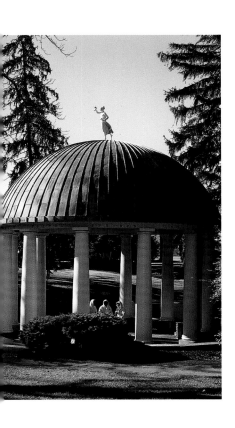

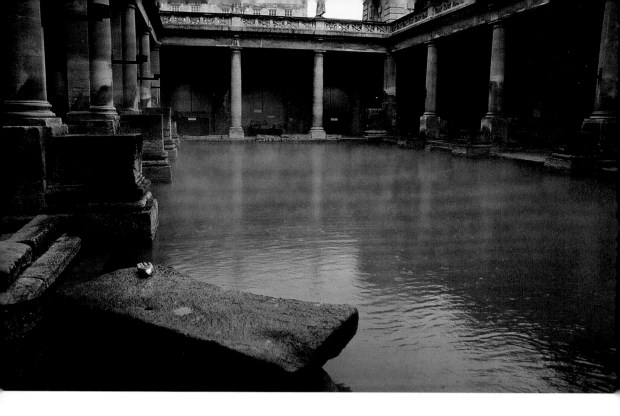

SPAS THROUGH THE AGES

A Barbarian warlord once asked a Roman emperor why he bathed once a day. "Alas," the emperor replied, "because I don't have time to bathe *twice* a day."

When this conversation took place, about two thousand years ago, the sacred nature of water was already an ancient idea. Water was the giver of life, a miraculous rejuvenator, a conduit to the divine. Throughout the world, mineral springs were not only great centers of healing, but religious sites for communing with gods, goddesses, and saints.

They were also the first spas.

The ancient Greeks were serious about their baths. Hippocrates, the father of modern medicine, recommended them to prevent disease. The bathhouses of Greece even had gymnasiums and lecture halls. But it was the Romans, with their great aqueducts and elaborate architecture, who turned spa life into an art. They loved a good massage, sauna, and whirlpool soak whenever they could get it, and their bathhouses were fitted with libraries, art galleries, and gymnasiums. Pliny the Elder estimated that by the first century A.D. there were nearly one thousand public bathhouses in Rome. The word *spa*, inscribed as graffiti on many ancient bathhouse walls, comes from the Latin phrase *sanitas per aquas*, which means "health through water." The Romans believed thermal mineral water to be good medicine for everything from gout to infertility.

The Roman spa, however, was far more than a place for a soak. Spas were a social destination where political debates laid the foundations for the great events of the time. The spas were also religious sites, complete with temples, and the Romans were experts at combining the spiritual with the decadent. The bathhouse was a place to give the opposite sex a look, and sometimes a good deal more. Before Emperor Hadrian banned coed bathing in 138 A.D., Roman spas were notorious as steamy cauldrons of adultery.

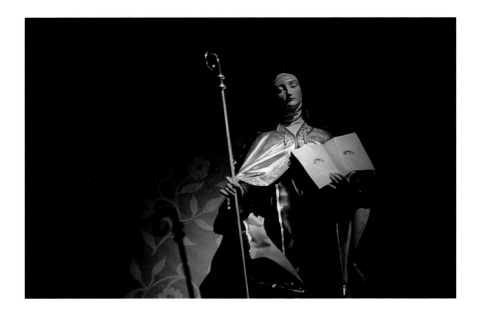

Roman bathhouses differed from spas of today in another way: food. Today's spa cuisine is a far cry from the tasteless, low-cal offerings of a few decades ago, but you certainly won't find sausage snacks, as in Roman times. The playwright Seneca complained that "the roaring babel" of sausage vendors was so loud, he could barely think. The Romans believed that bathing in the springs actually *increased* appetite, and would take to the waters after downing a huge meal to make room for another course. Emperor Commodus took up to eight baths a day for just this purpose.

But the Roman spa was a fitness center, too. Spa-goers played competitive sports on the bathhouse grounds and frequented fitness rooms, where they pumped iron and worked out using state-of-the-art burlap punching bags filled with flour. These jocks also annoyed Seneca. "I can hear them grunt as they strain, or pretend to, hissing and gasping as they expel their breath after holding it," he wrote.

Of course, as the Romans conquered the world around them, they spread their water-loving culture wherever they found a worthy mineral spring: Baden-Baden, Germany; Bath, England; Budapest, Hungary; and Spa, Belgium (where Roman coins have been found). Excavations of Roman ruins have revealed highly sophisticated plumbing, heating, and engineering systems, as well as gloriously ornate saunas and baths. Several of these sites were regarded as sacred for centuries prior to the Romans' arrival. The springs at Bath, for instance, had long been a holy place where the ancient Celts worshipped their water god, Sulis.

Even after the Roman Empire fell, hot-spring sites remained popular. Tales of miraculous cures perpetuated the belief that the waters were touched by the divine.

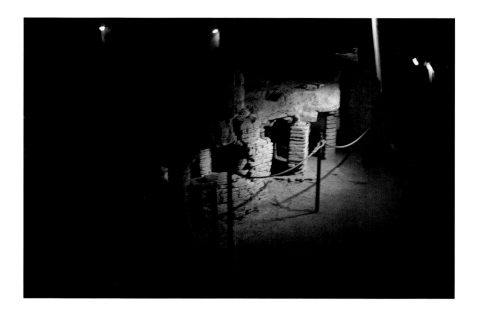

In Spa, Belgium, St. Remaclus was believed to have possessed the power to purify fountains and create springs. It was even thought that when an infertile woman placed her foot on a stone where the saint had left his imprint, she would become pregnant. During the Middle Ages, so many visitors flocked to the village's spring that a "cure tax" was levied.

A true renaissance of spa life began in the eighteenth century, when the hot-springs cities of Europe began reverting to their Roman-style roots. Perhaps the greatest of all was Bath, England. Here, renowned architect John Wood raised fairy-tale buildings shaped in crescents, circles, and squares. Boosted by publicity from the charismatic socialite Beau Nash, Bath attracted hordes of health-seeking tourists, from royalty to wannabes. "Taking the waters" became a most fashionable pastime. Visitors would spend the day soaking in the baths and drinking the thermal waters before an afternoon of high tea. Evening entertainment included ballroom dancing and gambling. The greatest artists and writers—Thomas Gainsborough, Charles Dickens, Jonathan Swift—visited, some finding rich material in the social scene. Jane Austen wrote of it in *Northanger Abbey* and Tobias Smollett lampooned it in *Humphry Clinker.*

By the nineteenth century, Baden-Baden had begun to replace Bath as the most fashionable spa destination in Europe. Some called it the summer capital of the Continent, drawing visitors such as Queen Victoria, Napoleon the Third, and a host of artists. Chopin and Balzac were frequent visitors, as well as Dostoyevsky, who spent his time gambling in the casinos.

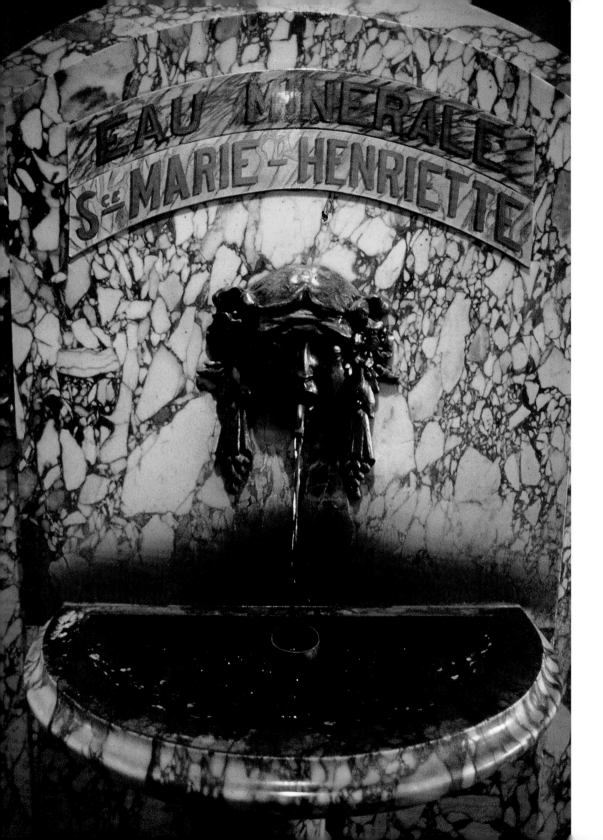

It was at this time, too, that the United States began developing a spa culture of its own. Places like Saratoga Springs, New York and Hot Springs, Arkansas—long regarded as powerful healing sites by Native Americans—drew a similarly varied lot of colorful characters. In its heydey, Hot Springs attracted U.S. presidents, including both Theodore and Franklin Roosevelt, notorious gangsters like Al Capone (he and his entourage would often rent out an entire floor of the Arlington Hotel), and sports legends such as Babe Ruth. Baseball magnate A. G. Spaulding brought his team here "to boil the alcohol microbes out of them." The town theater attracted Broadway plays and other high-quality acts from all over the country. Novelist Stephen Crane once wrote that Hot Springs was such a center of diversity "that no one need feel strange here."

In 1921, the forty-seven springs and surrounding oak-and-hickory-covered hills were designated a National Park. Hot Springs flourished until the mid-twentieth century when advancements in modern medicine made it seem obsolete. Today, the grand old Arlington Hotel, a favorite watering hole with two springs, still stands like a queen over "Bathhouse Row," an elaborate monument to the roaring, glamorous spa days of yore. The bathhouses, with their Italian marble, fountains of water gods, and stained-glass windows, were meant to invoke Rome at the height of its hedonistic glory. Only one remains open to the public for bathing, but the waters can be taken at a few of the hotels.

Today's spas have kept the best of the past, and discarded much of the rest. Most no longer claim to cure disease, but promise to help maintain health. Some have doctors and medical technology on-site. Recent scientific research cites massage, meditation. and other relaxation techniques as a way of reducing stress-related illness. Many of the cures that took place at the hot springs in the past have since been attributed to the rest, relaxation, and inspiration provided to visitors. (The minerals in the waters may have also aided digestion.)

Pioneers like Edmond and Deborah Szekely introduced the idea of exercise and healthy foods as guiding principles of a spa experience. The "health camp" they started in the 1940s, just past the California border in Mexico, would become the first modern spa in North America (see page 174). There, long before it was fashionable, they served fresh vegetarian food, grown with no pesticides. They also preached the importance of connecting with nature to put one's life in perspective.

And that is the basic formula for the spa of today: A beautiful environment to relieve stress; healthy food to nourish the body; and a focus on the relationship between body and mind. Spas are places to find both solitude and society. Places to change what doesn't work in life, and to celebrate what does.

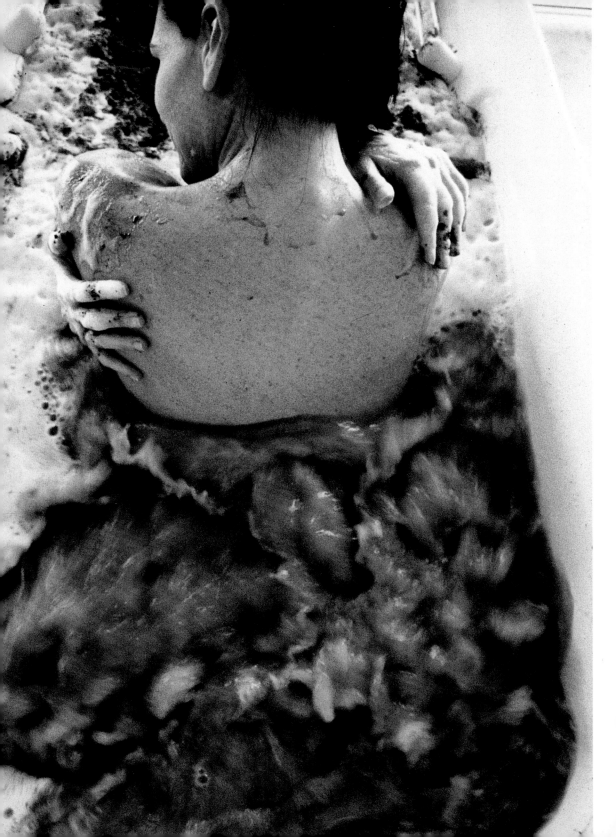

SPA FOOD

As you lie on a massage table, the smell of Christmas cookies lingers. A walnut, coconut, and vanilla scrub looks like cookie dough, but instead it's an exfoliant, concocted to make your skin as soft as butter-cream frosting.

More and more food is making its way into the treatment room. One would think this trend comes from a subconscious desire to eat. Can't have chocolate. Okay, let's slather it on. But the truth is, no one goes hungry at most spas today. Gone are the bland, the boiled, and the miniscule. Today we get filet mignon with low-fat sauces and gravies that rival their heavier ancestors; fresh herbs bursting with flavor, replacing some of the duties of salt; and luscious cheesecake made with low-fat ricotta and yogurt. Comfort food is also not a problem: While it's still hard to find truly rich-tasting macaroni and cheese, vegetable pizza and a tuna melt spa-style leave little to be desired.

The growing trend of using foods for body treatments does not stem from hungry desire, but from the enjoyment of the sensual, like a fine meal. A look at recent treatment fare reveals fruits (pineapple, mangoes, and pomegranates), as well as sweets (sugar, honey, and vanilla), and vegetables (ground corn and cucumbers), many of which are said to provide a rich supply of antioxidants to stave off those infamous free-radicals that deplete the skin of elasticity and youth. Other ingredients, such as milk and honey, have been known for their moisturizing benefits since Cleopatra's time. Now, of course, with recipes more sophisticated, you can have eggnog in place of milk. And what would a little indulgence be without coffee (exfoliant) and chocolate (moisturizer)?

A chocolate whirlpool bath (shown opposite at Kurotel in Brazil) is perhaps the ultimate fantasy for chocolate lovers. The enticing aroma of rich cocoa swirls through the air as white foam froths up around you like whipped cream. You sink in deeper and are tempted to take a sip. But don't do it; there's a spa dessert waiting for you somewhere.

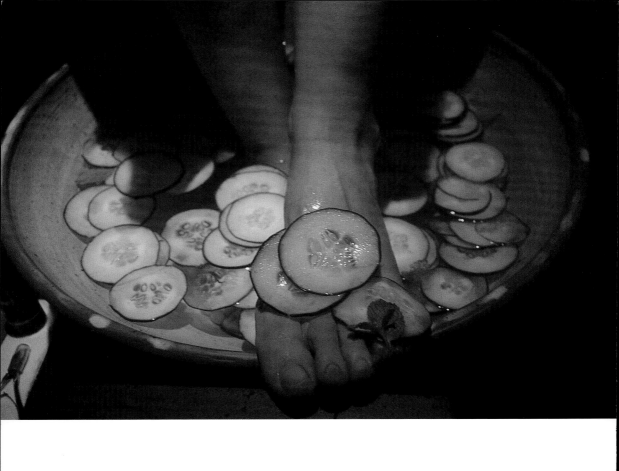
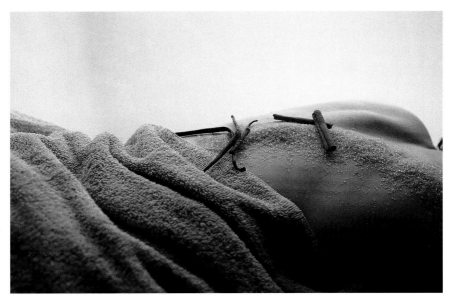

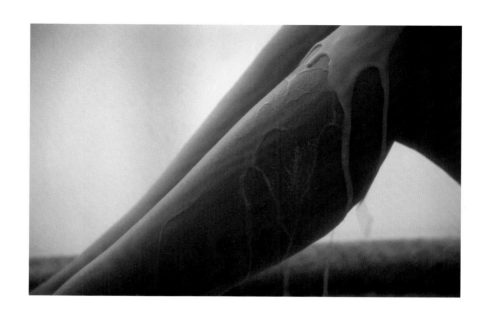

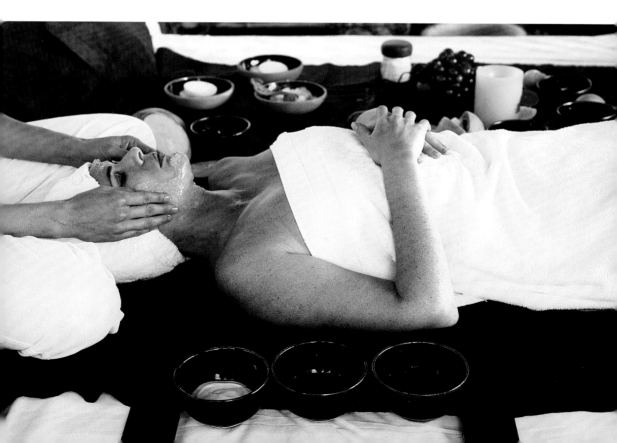

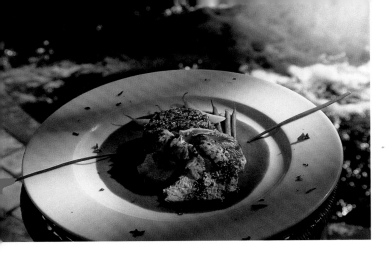

Himalayan Red Rice with Baby Vegetables in Asparagus Sauce with Braised Breast of Chicken

Presented by Miraval, Life in Balance Resort®
Yields 4 servings

HIMALAYAN RED RICE WITH APPLES AND ALMONDS
Yields 10 servings

2 1/2 cups vegetable stock
1 cup Himalayan red rice
1/2 cup chopped scallions
1 cinnamon stick
1 whole star anise
1 cup chopped Granny Smith apple (about 1 apple)
1 tablespoon toasted, chopped almond
1/8 teaspoon freshly ground black pepper
1/4 teaspoon sea salt

In a medium saucepan bring to a boil the vegetable stock, rice, scallions, cinnamon, and star anise. Reduce heat, and simmer for 40 minutes until rice starts to soften. Remove from heat and mix in apple, almond, pepper, and salt. Cover again and let rice steep for 5 more minutes. Fluff with a fork and serve.

Per serving (1/2 cup): Calories 90; Protein 2g; Total Fat 1g; Saturated Fat 0g; Carbohydrates 19g; Dietary Fiber 2g; Cholesterol 0mg; Sodium 65mg

ASPARAGUS SAUCE
Yields 3 cups

1/2 teaspoon extra virgin olive oil
1 cup chopped onion (about 1 large)
2 teaspoons minced fresh garlic
4 cups chopped asparagus stems (about 2 bunches)—save tops for garnish
1 teaspoon minced fresh ginger
3 cups vegetable stock
2 cups fresh spinach, stems removed and washed
1/4 cup cornstarch mixed with 1/4 cup vegetable stock
1/4 teaspoon sea salt
1/4 teaspoon freshly ground black pepper
1/4 teaspoon ground nutmeg

Heat a medium saucepan over medium heat and add olive oil to coat bottom of pan. Stir in onion, garlic, asparagus, and ginger and cook until onion has softened, about 5 minutes. Pour in stock and simmer for 3 minutes. (Do not overcook asparagus; you want it to be bright green.) Add spinach and simmer for 2 minutes.

Carefully ladle asparagus mixture into a blender and process until smooth. Strain the purée through a colander lined with cheesecloth or through a fine mesh sieve. Pour the strained mixture back into the saucepan and bring to a low boil. Mix in cornstarch mixture and cook, stirring constantly, until sauce thickens and coats the back of a spoon. Season with the salt, pepper, and nutmeg.

Use the sauce immediately or cool down in an ice bath. Store in an airtight container for up to 1 week in the refrigerator or freeze for about 1 month.

Per serving (1/4 cup): Calories 50; Protein 2g; Total Fat 2g; Saturated Fat 0g; Carbohydrates 8g; Dietary Fiber 2g; Cholesterol 0mg; Sodium 65mg

BRAISED BREAST OF CHICKEN
Yields 4 servings

1/8 teaspoon extra virgin olive oil
4 (4-ounce) skinless chicken breasts
1/2 teaspoon sea salt
1/4 teaspoon ground black pepper
3/4 cup vegetable stock

Heat a large sauté pan over high flame and add olive oil to coat bottom of pan. Season chicken breasts with salt and pepper. Place chicken breasts in pan and sear on one side until brown. Turn chicken pieces, deglaze with 3/4 cup of vegetable stock, and simmer 3 minutes until chicken is cooked throughout.

Asparagus spears, 2 bunches
(use tops for entrée and stems for sauce)
Steamed assorted vegetables
1 teaspoon chopped mixed herbs
1 cup asparagus sauce

To serve: Ladle 1/4 cup of sauce in the center of each plate. Using a 1/2-cup measuring cup or mold, mound the rice in the center of each plate. Toss the steamed vegetables with the herbs and arrange beside rice. Slice chicken and fan over rice.

Per serving: Calories 330; Protein 33g; Total Fat 4g; Saturated Fat 0.5g; Carbohydrates 43g; Dietary Fiber 6g; Cholesterol 65mg; Sodium 540mg

Hot Asian Soba Noodles, Prawns & Shiitake Mushrooms with Curry Coconut Yam Sauce

Presented by The Golden Door®
Yields 4 servings

1 teaspoon olive oil or canola oil spray
1 tablespoon shallot, peeled and thinly sliced
1 teaspoon ginger, minced
1 clove garlic, thinly sliced
1 stalk lemongrass, cut into three pieces, smashed
1 small (about 6-ounce) yam, peeled and sliced
1 cup chicken stock or water
1/2 teaspoon Thai curry paste, or to taste
14 ounces low-fat coconut milk
12 ounces (about 16) prawns, peeled and de-veined
2 teaspoons dark sesame oil
1 tablespoon garlic, minced
3 tablespoons low-sodium soy sauce
4 ounces soba noodles
4 cups (one bunch) spinach, washed
8 whole shiitake mushrooms, stems removed, quartered
1/4 cup dry white wine or chicken stock, warm to hot
1 teaspoon ginger root, grated and the juice extracted
1 tablespoon lime juice
1/4 cup scallions, sliced thin on the bias
2 tablespoons chopped chives
1 whole lime cut into wedges

Lightly spray olive or canola oil onto bottom of heavy saucepan and place over medium heat. Stir together sliced shallot, minced ginger, sliced garlic, and smashed lemongrass. Add sliced yam and stir 1 to 2 minutes.

Add 1 cup chicken stock. Add Thai curry paste to taste and simmer 10 to 15 minutes. Add low-fat coconut milk and simmer an additional 20 to 25 minutes until reduced by half.

Remove lemongrass stalk and let mixture cool 15 to 20 minutes. Transfer mixture to blender and blend until smooth. Return to pan and keep warm.

In a nonreactive pan, combine the cleaned shrimp, sesame oil, garlic, and soy sauce. Marinate, covered, for 30 minutes, in the refrigerator.

Meanwhile, bring a medium-sized pot of lightly salted water to a boil. Add soba noodles and simmer for 5 minutes, or until noodles are just soft. Drain and put aside.

Heat a nonstick skillet over medium heat, add cleaned spinach, and cook, stirring often, until spinach just begins to wilt but remains vivid green in color. Stir in the drained soba noodles and keep warm.

Spray a medium nonstick pan with the olive/canola spray and place over medium-high heat. Add prawns, shiitake mushrooms, and any remaining marinade, and saute for 3 to 5 minutes, stirring often. Add 1/4 cup dry white wine or chicken stock. Add ginger juice and return to simmer for 1 to 2 minutes, until the prawns are firm.

Squeeze 1 tablespoon lime juice into warm yam sauce and spoon approximately 4 tablespoons of sauce into center of each of 4 large plates. Mound spinach and soba noodles in the center of sauce. Place prawns and shiitake mushrooms around soba noodles and sprinkle with scallions and chives. Serve immediately, garnished with lime wedges.

Yields 1 1/4 cups

Per serving: Calories 307; Protein 25g; Total Fat 4g (12% calories from fat); Carbohydrates 45g; Cholesterol 129mg; Sodium 1368mg

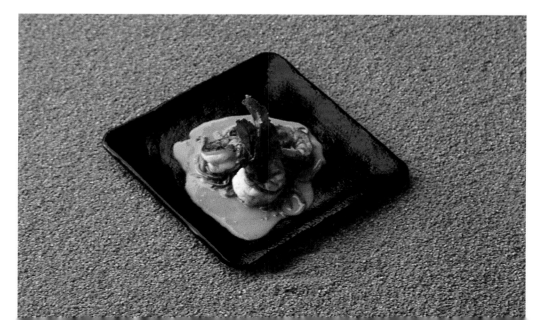

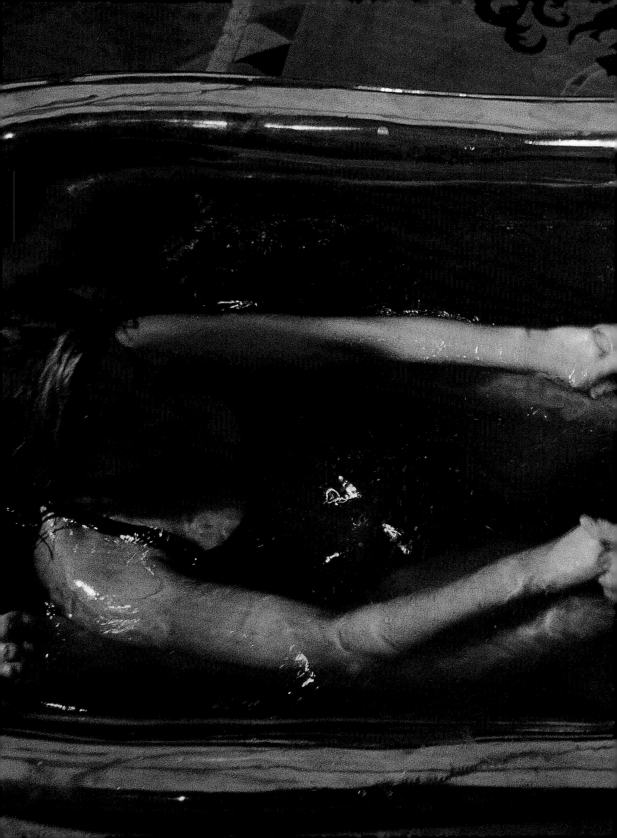

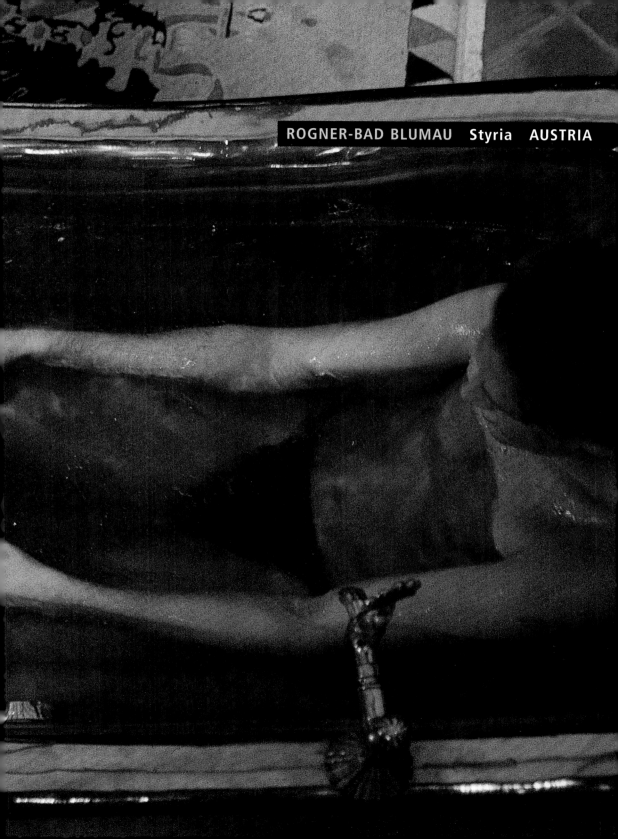

ROGNER-BAD BLUMAU Styria AUSTRIA

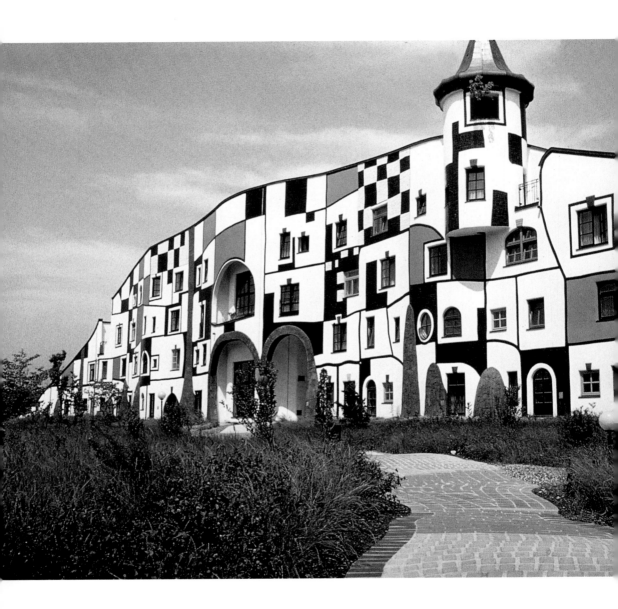

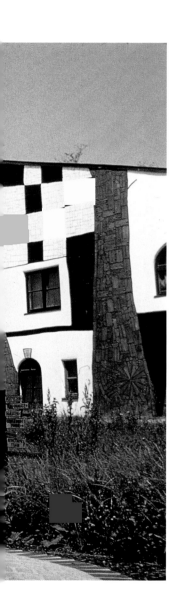

ROGNER-BAD BLUMAU, STYRIA, AUSTRIA

Austria's famed architect Friedensreich Hundertwasser has created at Blumau a whimsical world that looks like a stage set for a sequel to *The Wizard of Oz*. From the outside, the walls resemble accordion divider-screens, ready to blow over with the first strong gust of wind. But apparently they're solid enough, for they've stood since 1997. Odder yet, grass has been planted on the roof, helping this man-made fantasyland to blend in with the lush countryside of southeastern Austria.

Hundertwasser, a painter as well as an architect, decried straight lines as "godless," claiming that they rarely appear in nature. All architectural details are circular and no window is the same size or shape, giving visitors a constant sense of movement and, at times, an Alice-falling-through-the-looking-glass feeling. The rooms have been described as "modern-day Fred Flintstone," with clean, Scandanavian-style furnishings. Many European sophisticates say that if you surrender to the creative atmosphere, you will begin to feel a wonderful childlike joy.

Even if you sense no joy in the architecture, you are sure to find it in the abundant thermal springs. They were discovered in the 1970s by an oil company drilling for gas, and they are now the main attraction. One can swim from the outdoor pool to the indoor pool, where footbridges arch over the waterways (a little slice of Venice), sometimes ending in a cul-de-sac with underwater benches.

Despite its funhouse design, the spa is a place of serious aspiration. Like the architecture, treatments are innovative and creative. The hay bath (yes, as in horses) is especially popular. It's more like a "hay cocoon," as hay (steam-heated to eliminate allergens) is layered over the body, helping you to sweat out toxins. It is recommended for soothing achy muscles and improving circulation. Also offered are past-life regression therapy and sound therapy, in which you lie on a special table suspended above a fifty-stringed instrument. The vibrations from the sound are supposed to balance the body's aura, or energy field. Tibetan bowls are also placed along the body's chakras, and a wand brings their various tones to a crescendo. While they may not balance chakras, they produce profound relaxation.

The spa also has an elaborate array of saunas and steam baths, from Finnish to Turkish to Roman. The "aroma grotto" features an illuminated hologram of the rain forest, with a citrus scent and recorded bird songs piped in. And what would a free-spirited Austrian resort be without a nudist colony? The spa has an 8,000 square-foot island tucked away behind the sauna area where one is welcome to soak up some rays au naturel.

If you tire of lounging around naked, take the two-hour drive to Vienna, where you can visit the innumerable world-famous museums—including one devoted to Hundertwasser, which critics lovingly call "every bit as bizarre" as the spa.

THIS SPA IS FOR YOU IF you're looking for something quirky and different, but with a Continental flare.

THIS SPA IS NOT FOR YOU IF you desire traditional European luxury and have no interest in a hotel that could have been designed by Andy Warhol.

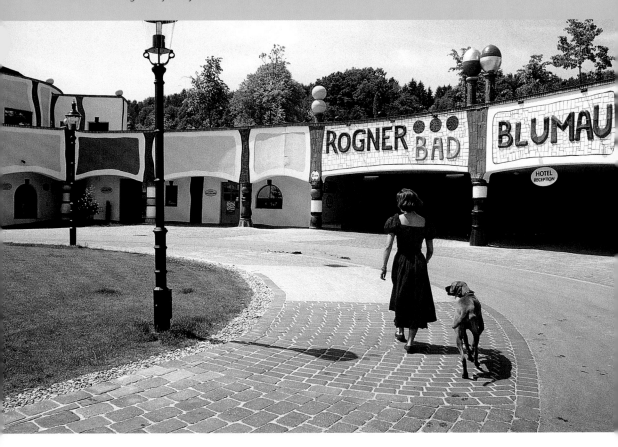

PRICE $$

ROOMS 247
Basic, clean & pleasant.

FOOD
Made with fresh produce from nearby organic farms. Includes regional and gourmet Austrian fare, vegetarian selections and low-fat cuisine. Local treat is healthy pumpkin-seed oil, great on salads.

OUTSTANDING TREATMENTS
Aphrodite Bath (with saffron, honey and mare's milk); Hay Bath; and Sound Therapy.

ACTIVITIES
Visiting a working dairy farm; Horseback Riding; Tennis; Hiking; Biking; and Hot-Air Ballooning. Golf Courses nearby.

CLASSES
Aqua-Jogging and Spinning (both in German).

NEARBY ATTRACTIONS
Vienna (check out KunstHausWien, the museum devoted to the spa's architect); Boat Ride on the Danube.

FOR CHILDREN
Free childcare for ages 4–12.

CONFERENCE SPACE
Six conference rooms.

GETTING THERE
A 2-hour drive from Vienna airport.

ADDRESS
A-8283
Bad Blumau 100
Austria

T 43-3383-5100-0   **F** 43-3383-5100-808   **E** spa.blumau@rogner.com   **W** www.blumau.com

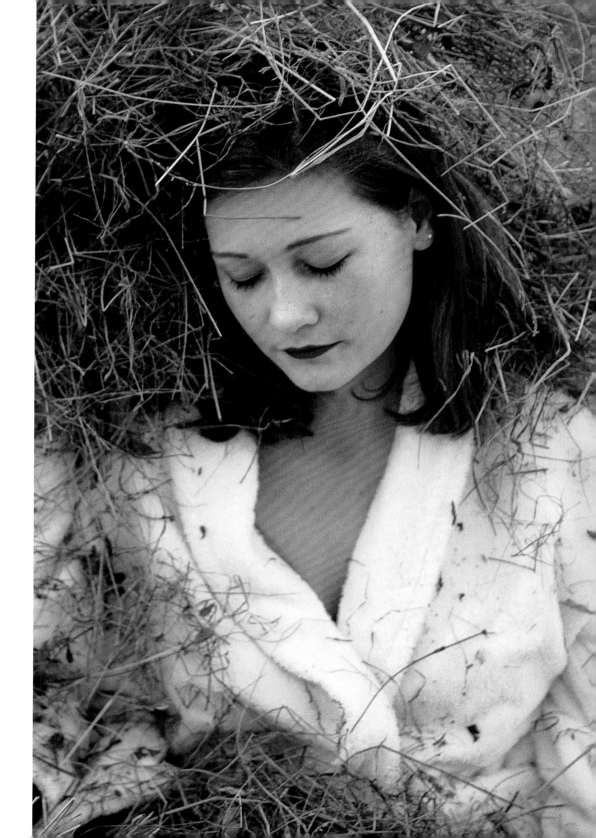

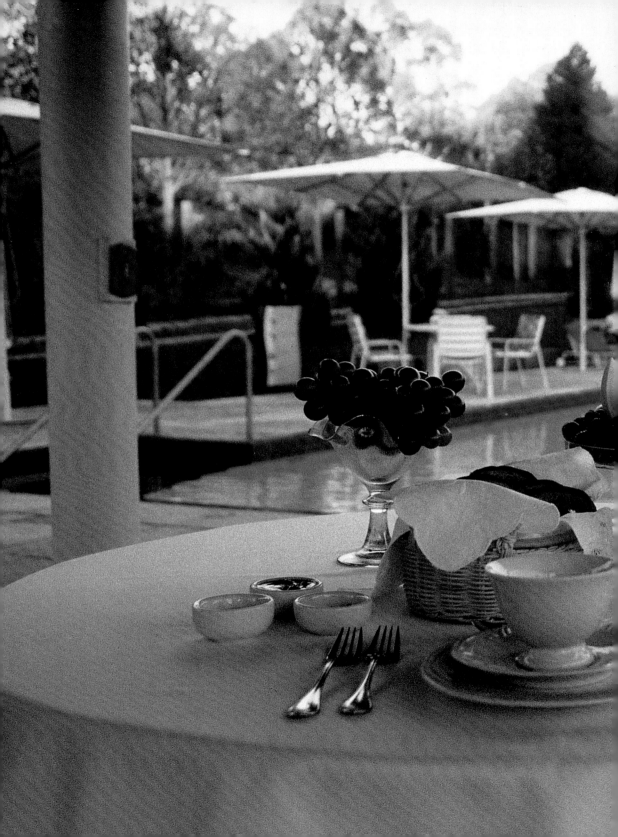

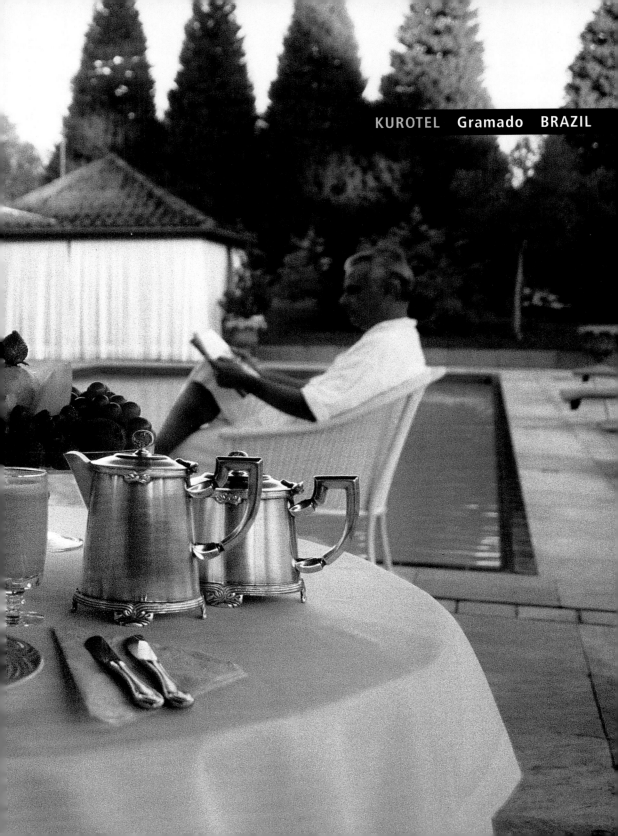

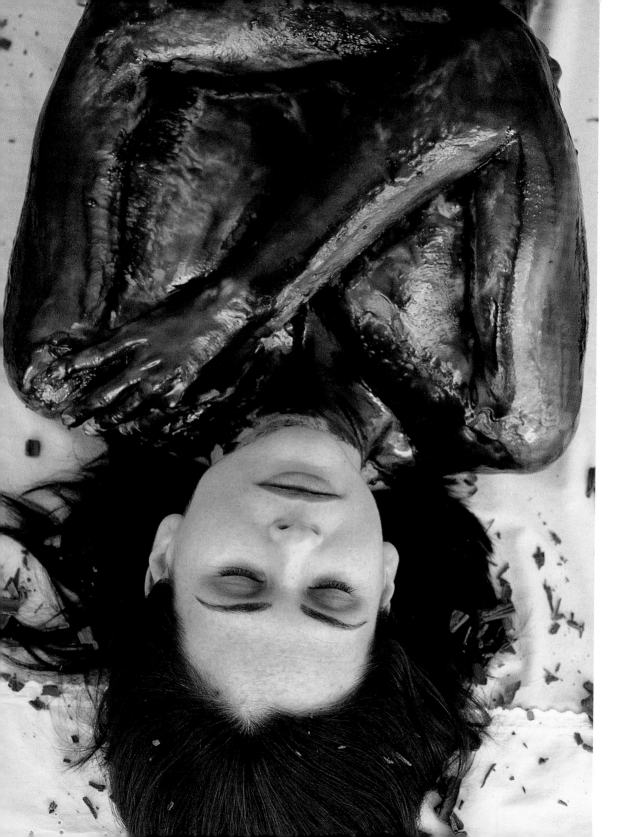

KUROTEL, GRAMADO, BRAZIL

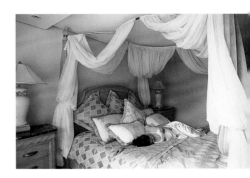

"Thank you! I love you! I want to kiss you!"

These are the three English expressions Fernando knows. Nonetheless, Fernando, the excitable samba-aerobics instructor at Kurotel, will scream them at the top of his lungs with a huge smile on his face once he finds out you're an American. This may sound annoying, but when the samba beat grabs hold of you, you'll be swept away by the music and might even find yourself shouting right back.

Fernando and the rest of the charming, enthusiastic staff at Kurotel are one of this destination's great draws. Everyone seems to love having an American around, relishing the opportunity to hone their English and to inquire how things are going up North. Solo travelers will not be lonely. Not only does the staff look after you, but Kurotel is a spot that attracts some of Brazil's most famous artists and politicians, many of whom speak English.

If you're thinking of visiting Rio (about an hour's plane ride away), and want to feel good in a string bikini, this is the perfect place to go beforehand. When you first arrive, you confer with a spa doctor who will review your medical history and discuss any goals you may have for your stay. For instance, mention those few pounds you would like to lose and the doc may put you on an eight-hundred-calorie-a-day diet. I decided to give it a try, at least for a few days. Forget the string bikini—I just wanted to zip up my trousers without groaning.

The first day, I lined up for my afternoon snack, salivating for a yogurt mousse. Like many spas outside of the United States, this one is somewhat behind the times when it comes to spa food; they still serve meager portions, and what's offered is rather tasteless, though beautifully arranged. On the second day, I decided to up my caloric intake to a whopping eleven hundred per day, and I actually could taste the potatoes (they had a creamy, cheesy sauce). Ironically, on the third day, after admiring, but not really tasting, the food (mostly vegetable purée soups, chicken, and grilled fish), I was told the doctor wanted to see me.

"Sit down, Madame," Dr. Eduardo Melnick said, with a look of such concern that I began to worry I might be seriously ill.

"I am afraid," he said slowly, "that you've gained a gram since yesterday." Had I gone to town, eaten some chocolate? (I had not, though the town of Gramado is famous for its chocolate.) Maybe, I said, it was the second portion of potatoes I'd had at dinner last night. Dr. Eduardo clucked his tongue and carefully examined my records. He looked at the results from a test I'd previously undergone that had used a high-tech machine (of which the spa is very proud), a sort of fat-measuring X-ray machine that detects just where in the body excess weight is distributed. Too much weight in the middle can signal potential heart problems.

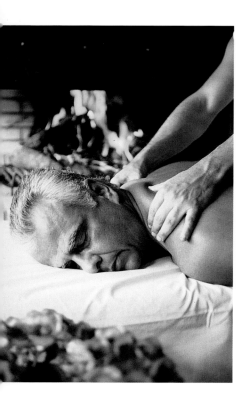

"I see you don't need to lose weight for health reasons," he said. "But if you really want to lose some weight in the next few days, maybe we should put you back on eight hundred calories." We compromised at nine hundred.

The following days were some of the most enjoyable I've ever had on such a strict health regimen. Kurotel is its own cozy world of elegance and ease. The exercise room has a view of the lush tropical vegetation common to this southern mountain region. Each day's activities were laid out for me the night before, based on my goals: treadmill, aqua-aerobics (very easy to follow even in Portuguese), and a Kneipp treatment—a walk along a water path whose temperature changes from cold to warm (believed to help circulation and stimulate the immune system).

The spa dedicates an entire wing to the Stress Control Center, which sounds Orwellian (some of the technology is a bit futuristic), but is actually quite peaceful and interesting. First I tried a biofeedback session. The therapist hooked me up to machines that measure heart rate and perspiration, and asked me questions designed to cause stress—she tested my memory by having me count backwards from one thousand while playing music interrupted by loud static. When my stress level went up, she had me take a deep breath. Once I took a breath, my levels fell, indicating that I manage stress pretty effectively. This surprised me, but was an encouraging sign. I realized that I must utilize the breath more often.

Several rooms in the Stress Control Center contain "float" machines, such as the revolving NASA chair that simulates zero gravity. It comes with a headset offering music and a lightshow. You may tire of these contraptions once the novelty wears off, but they're worth squeezing in between workouts.

The body treatments are also novel. You can soak in a chocolate bath, or in a wine *kur* (said to be beneficial due to the antioxidant properties of grapes), or try the rain forest scrub with *cupuacu*, a fruit found in the Amazon region that looks like a kiwi, also containing antioxidant nutrients. Each treatment room is a little world unto itself, much like rooms in Japanese hotels designed to cater to individual fantasies. The wine kur room is decorated with wood barrels and plastic vines hung from the ceiling; the rain forest room features local flora and a stone shower; the chocolate room is paneled in dark wood and has a cozy fireplace.

The chocolate bath treatment is a favorite. The tub jets whir, white foam rises to the top, and it's like soaking in a giant cup of hot cocoa topped with whipped cream. I was so hungry on my nine hundred calories that I considered taking a sip. The benefits of chocolate go way beyond the taste and aroma, however; it's truly a wonderful emollient. Afterwards, I couldn't remember my skin ever feeling so soft. By the time I got to Rio, I was as velvet as a Hershey's Kiss, four pounds lighter, and walked to a samba beat.

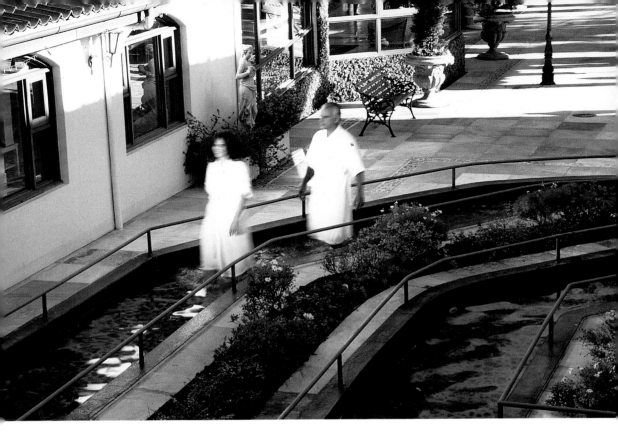

PRICE $$

ROOMS 35
Elegantly appointed.
The Executive Suites
have large rooms and
a common area with
Internet access.

FOOD
The main restaurant serves
good, though slightly
bland, low-fat food
cooked with fresh produce
from its own gardens. The
amount of food served
depends upon personal
goals determined at the
beginning of your stay. If
you're not trying to lose
weight, your choices
increase, as does the
amount of sauce used,
which, alas, is the only
thing that seems to
improve taste. No
alcohol is served.

**OUTSTANDING
TREATMENTS**
Chocolate Bath;
Chocolate Fondue; and
Rain Forest Scrub.

ACTIVITIES
Horseback Riding and
Golf nearby.

CLASSES
Aqua- and Samba-
Aerobics; Body Pump;
and Weight Training
(all in Portuguese).

FOR CHILDREN
Special program for new
mothers and their babies,
featuring private cabanas
and much pampering.

NEARBY ATTRACTIONS
The small town of
Gramado, famous for its
chocolate. Gramado is also
a great place to shop for
good-quality Brazilian
shoes at bargain prices.

GETTING THERE
An hour's drive from Porto
Alegre airport (connect in
Rio or São Paulo).

ADDRESS
Rua Nacoes Unidas, 553
PO Box 65
CEP 95670-000 Gramado
Rio do Sul, Brazil

T 55-54-286-2133   **F** 55-54-286-1203   **E** reservations@kurotel.com.br   **W** www.kurotel.com

THIS SPA IS FOR YOU IF you want to lose a few pounds to look great in Rio.

THIS SPA IS NOT FOR YOU IF you hate a disciplined weight-loss regimen.

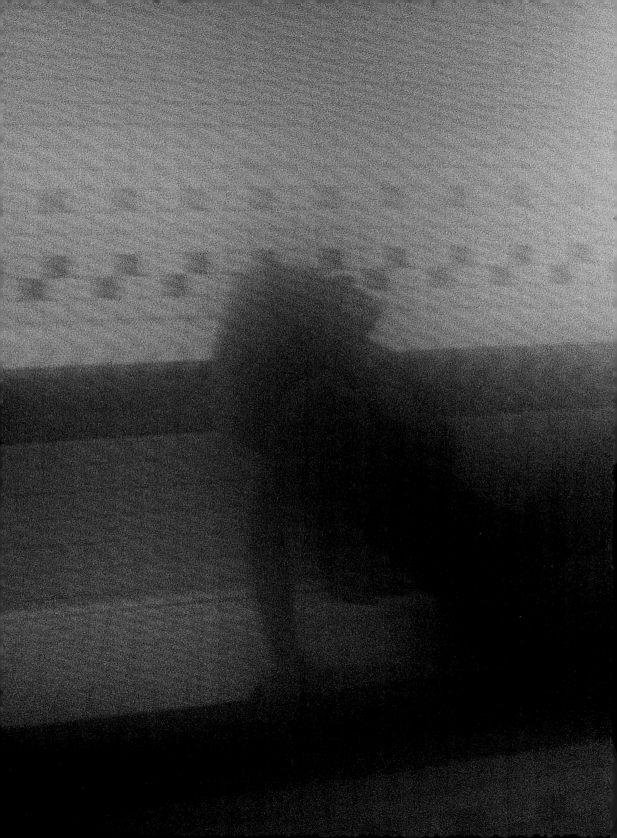

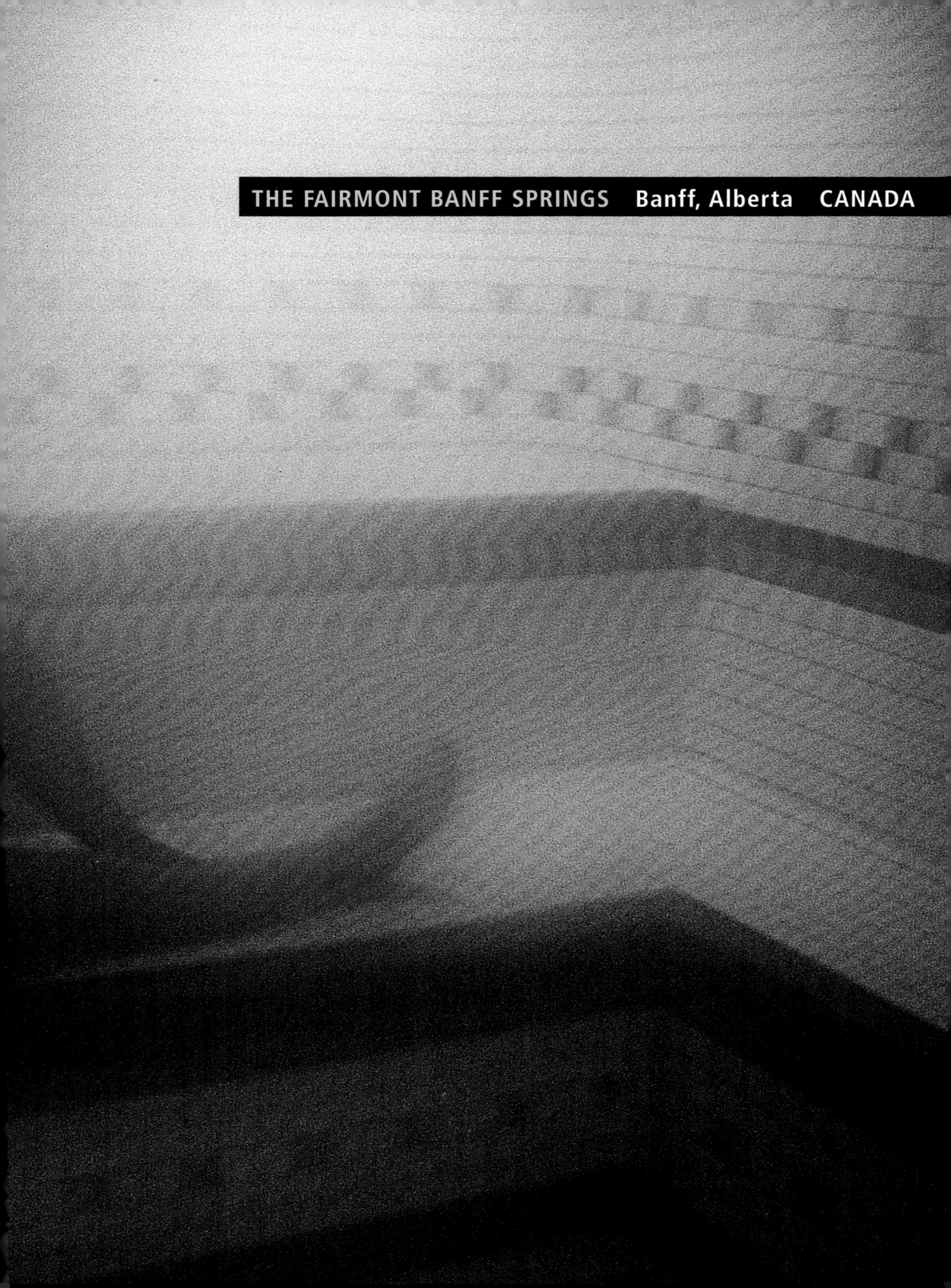

THE FAIRMONT BANFF SPRINGS Banff, Alberta CANADA

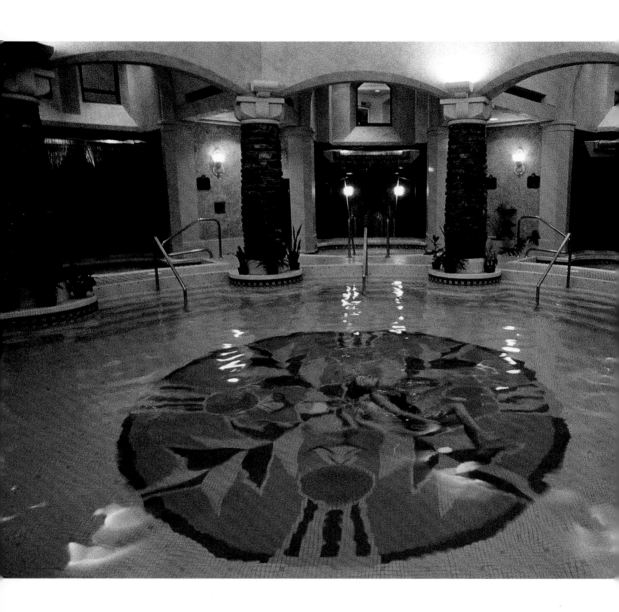

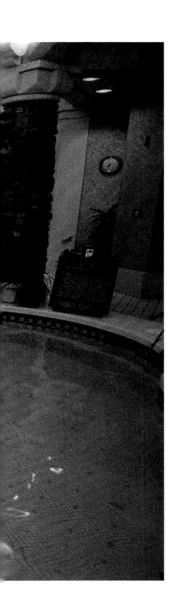

THE FAIRMONT BANFF SPRINGS, BANFF, ALBERTA, CANADA

Magnificently set in the glacier-capped Canadian Rockies, this castle dedicated to opulence, surrounded by nothing but alpine forest, appears dropped from the sky as if by magic. Its turreted eminence, which can be described as Scottish baronial meets French château, seems out of place in such pristine wilderness. Yet somehow it works.

This is a place where one can sip afternoon tea after horseback riding or order grilled ostrich medallions for dinner after heli-hiking. And it's a place where elk roam nonchalantly across a twenty-seven-hole golf course.

When Banff Springs was built in 1888 by Cornelius Van Horne, vice president of the Canadian Pacific Railroad, the 770-room fairy-tale castle was the largest hotel in the world. Van Horne's intention was to attract passengers to the railroad, and he figured that if he couldn't export the scenery, he would import the tourists.

The scenery in this part of the world is so spectacular that it looks surreal. The glacial lakes are a blue that exudes an eerie, otherworldly glow, and the meadows are so green, they're essentially iridescent. The mountains, sculpted gargantuan fortresses, are the most splendid in nature's museum, set against the sky and reflected perfectly and precisely in the still, glacial waters.

One of the most comfortable spots to take in the scenery is the thermal mineral springs at the base of Sulphur Mountain. Once you get past the sulfur smell (which doesn't take long), you can experience the floating bliss of the water as you gaze upon a view that makes you feel as if you're perched on the edge of the world, looking out toward heaven. Most visitors like to hike up the mountain (or take a gondola ride) and then hit the pools on the way down.

Because the Canadian park system conserves the springs at Sulphur Mountain, the hotel imports its mineral water from a town in Hungary, where the water is recognized as having healing properties (aiding circulation and the immune system as well as sore muscles and joints). Another advantage of the Hungarian water is that it has no sulfurous smell.

The spa's four indoor pools allow one to stay warm (it can get pretty cold in the Canadian wilderness once you step out of those thermal pools) and still retain the benefit of feeling close to nature. Floor-to-ceiling windows offer a view of the snowcapped Rockies as you revel in a cascading waterfall that massages your back. As an added perk, the main pool has an underwater sound system, providing a sound track for this most dramatic of nature shows.

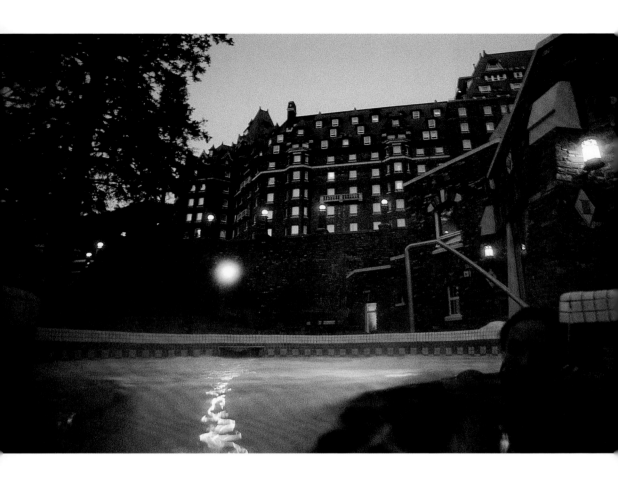

PRICE $$$

ROOMS 771
Elegantly appointed.

FOOD
Twelve restaurants
serving everything from
Italian to Japanese, and
grilled bison, venison, and
pheasant. Also available:
a pub, wine bar, bistro,
and spa restaurant.

**OUTSTANDING
TREATMENTS**
Wildflower Body Polish
and Rockies Rehydration
(includes an algae and
aloe vera wrap with hand,
neck, and foot massage).

CLASSES
Aerobics; Aqua-Aerobics;
and Yoga.

ACTIVITIES
27-hole Golf Course
(frequented by elk and
mule deer); Tennis;
Horseback Riding; Hiking;
Heli-Hiking; four Downhill
Ski areas; Cross-Country
Skiing; Snowshoeing;
Dogsledding; Skating; Ice
Fishing; Whitewater
Rafting; and Canoeing.

CONFERENCE SPACE
76,000 square feet of
meeting space.

GETTING THERE
A 90-minute drive from
Calgary airport.

ADDRESS
405 Spray Avenue
Banff, Alberta TIL 1J4

T 800-404-1772   **F** 403-762-5755   **E** bshreservations@fairmont.com   **W** www.willowstream.com

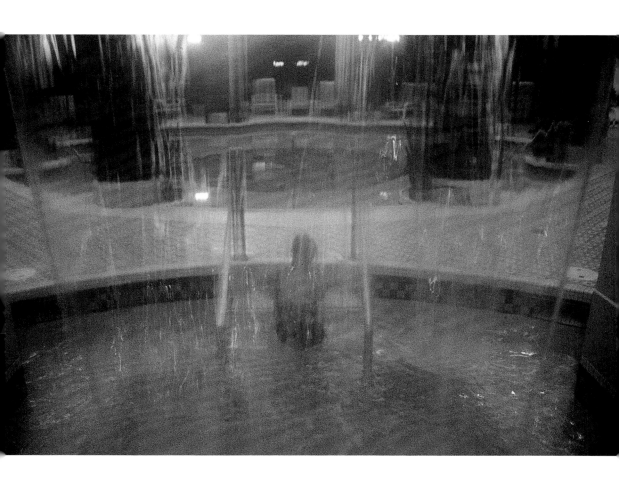

THIS SPA IS FOR YOU IF you love the great outdoors and some luxury to go with it.
THIS SPA IS NOT FOR YOU IF you prefer to experience the rugged outdoors in a more rustic and personal setting.

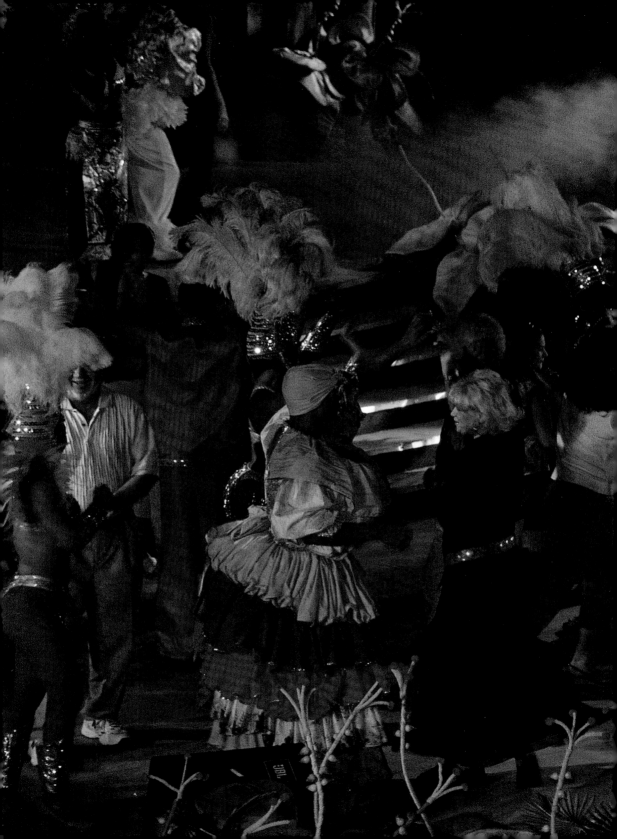

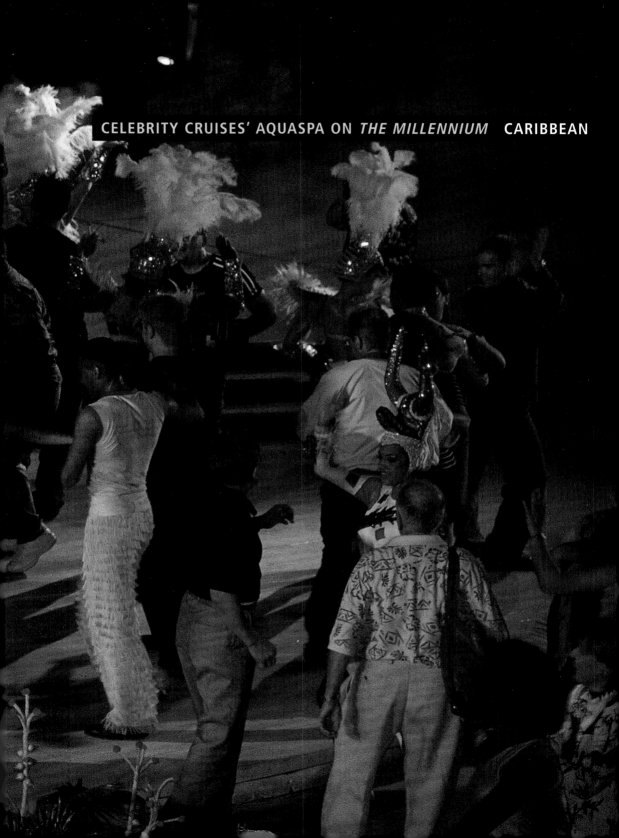

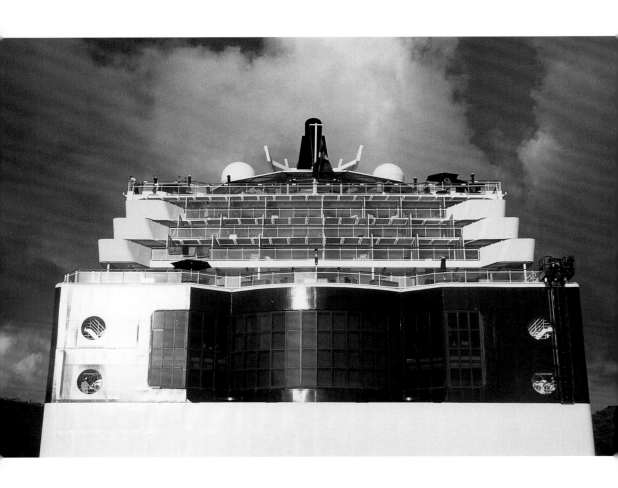

CELEBRITY CRUISES' AQUASPA ON *THE MILLENNIUM,* CARIBBEAN

The massage therapist's thumbs are pressing on my cheekbones in the delicate foreplay ritual that sometimes precedes a facial. She has long acrylic nails, like tiny humped antlers, but somehow she manages never to graze the surface of my skin. She presses four fingers from each hand to each side of my face and tugs, as if performing a face-lift. I'm getting the Japanese Silk Booster Facial, which includes a protein-serum silk mask reputed to take years off your appearance. Afterwards, she presses all ten of her acrylic-capped fingers over my scalp, and I am in ecstasy. My entire body relaxes as my muscles are rocked, soothed, and kneaded. It's not just the therapist causing this sensation—as I open my eyes, there it is: the ocean spreading itself before me, an undulating bed of water and foam.

Spas and cruises go together like...well, ships and water. My therapist that day, Claire Prior, is an instructor for Steiner, Ltd, a London-based company that staffs seaborne spas. The company's partner, Elemis, supplies the beauty products and treatments. On the modern cruise, shuffleboard just doesn't cut it anymore, and no ship gets built without adding a spa. Any treatment can be enhanced by the gentle rocking of the sea; you float in a beautiful, peaceful, alpha state, cocooned in the womb-like hull of the mama-ship, where even a facial feels like a full-body massage.

Celebrity Cruises' *Millennium* ship is one of its newest and, measuring 965 feet and weighing-in at 91,000 tons, it also boasts the largest spa-at-sea. With three restaurants, two theaters, and a casino on board, who would think you'd even notice the ocean? Linda Troeller, this book's photographer, definitely noticed: She tugged nervously at her acupressure wristbands before we even boarded the ship. "You're not even gonna feel it move," I reassured her. I told myself this as well. But once the engine roared out of the Fort Lauderdale port, we both turned green and wobbled to the medical center on Deck 1 for a supply of Bonine. Linda held out to see if the acupressure bands worked (they did) but I took enough Bonine to get high, and actually began enjoying the rolling waves. That evening, Linda and I sat in the nine-hundred-seat theater waving our piña coladas to the Celebrity performers' rendition of "One Singular Sensation." "See?" I whispered to Linda. "Can't even feel it moving."

The Millennium carries some two thousand passengers, so you may feel overwhelmed at times. But with a staff of close to a thousand, the service is excellent; room attendants act almost as personal butlers, smiling and greeting you as if they would take it personally if you didn't have fun.

The only time the crowd got a bit raucous was on the pool deck. When the band wasn't playing a reggae tune, an announcer would jump onstage and grab the microphone, trying to fill the dead air with forced joviality. (Some people seem to think you can't have fun unless you're downing shots and making lots of noise.) One afternoon I swooped in on a deck chair (the ship's policy is first-come, first-served, which eliminates the ugly practice of people lining up at 6 A.M. to reserve seats) and strategically placed it in just the right corner for a meditation on the azure ocean. Feeling the glow of the sun wash over me, I was jarred suddenly from my reverie by the booming voice of an MC. "Okay! It's time for our King of *The Millennium* contest!" Four male contestants bellowed like Tarzan and sang their favorite love songs a cappella. Alan, a senior citizen from New Jersey, sang "My Way" humorously off-key, and was crowned the winner.

There's always the lower deck to escape to. Even better, splurge for a stateroom with a private veranda and a view of the sea. The best thing about a cruise is the diversity found encapsulated in one vessel. You can wander downstairs to catch an auction of Picasso and Chagall prints, or roll the dice at the craps table in the casino. You can head straight from the pulsing beat of steel drums and greased

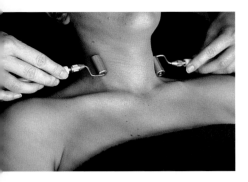

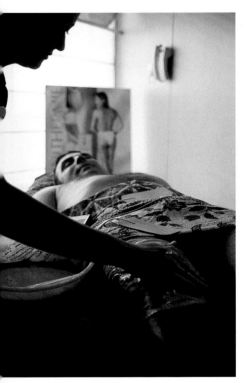

bodies at the pool to the quiet, cosseted world of white robes and wind chimes at the spa.

The moment you set foot into the spa's hushed, soothing, purple rooms, lavender oil permeates the air and the sound of the waves relaxes you. The fitness room, with floor-to-ceiling views, is quieter than the pool area. Most treatment rooms also have sea views, and at times you feel like you're right on the ocean, gliding as if on a magic-raft ride. The spa has a contraption called the "alpha capsule," which looks a bit like an amusement-park spaceship ride. As you lie in the capsule, it's supposed to produce alpha waves to help the body relax. But for the money ($35 for twenty-five minutes), you're better off getting an hour-long massage.

For those who crave neither the raucous outdoor pool party nor the hushed serenity of the treatment rooms, there is the thalassotherapy pool, which is set under a sunroof. Here you'll find the spa cafe discreetly tucked away, serving excellent low-fat meals and desserts all day until 8 P.M.

Food orgies are the stuff of cruise ships. Sit-down lunches, Tex-Mex buffets, Chinese lunches, midnight buffets (with pastries and frosted cakes), and after-dinner hors d'oeuvres in the nightclub are legendary cruise accoutrements. Your selection is limited only between the hours of 5 P.M., when tea ends, and the first seating for dinner, at 6 P.M. Between those hours one can choose from either the spa menu or the "carb menu"—pizza, French fries, or a hamburger. I sampled both and found the spa meals to be much tastier than the carbo-load. Much of the food on *The Millennium* is rather bland—the hamburger lacked that charcoal-grilled flavor, and the pizza was abundantly gloppy, with just a hint of tomato sauce. Choose the more interesting spa food—cold poached salmon, fruit salad, and tapioca pie—and avoid the seven extra pounds gained by the average passenger in a week. A sushi bar is another source of low-fat meals and the main dining room accommodates special menu requests.

However, don't expect to *lose* weight. It's impossible to avoid food—it's everywhere, all beautifully displayed. Few will be able to resist the colorful cookies and profiteroles that wink at you as you make your way to the pool. Part of the fun of such an array is trying a little bit of everything—if you don't like something, you move on to the next selection. The key phrase here is "little bit." A few not-so-spa-inclined passengers eat like they're stocking up for the winter, piling Tex-Mex volcanoes of food on their plates, constructing mountains of spareribs upon mounds of mashed potatoes. My most decadent act: consuming dinner, straight through to dessert (tasted four of them) before stumbling upon the sushi bar later that evening.

When it's time to exercise, try snorkeling or hiking at some of the ports-of-call. Casa de Campo in the Dominican Republic was our first stop, and it offered the opportunity for either a horseback ride or a brief walk around a replica of a

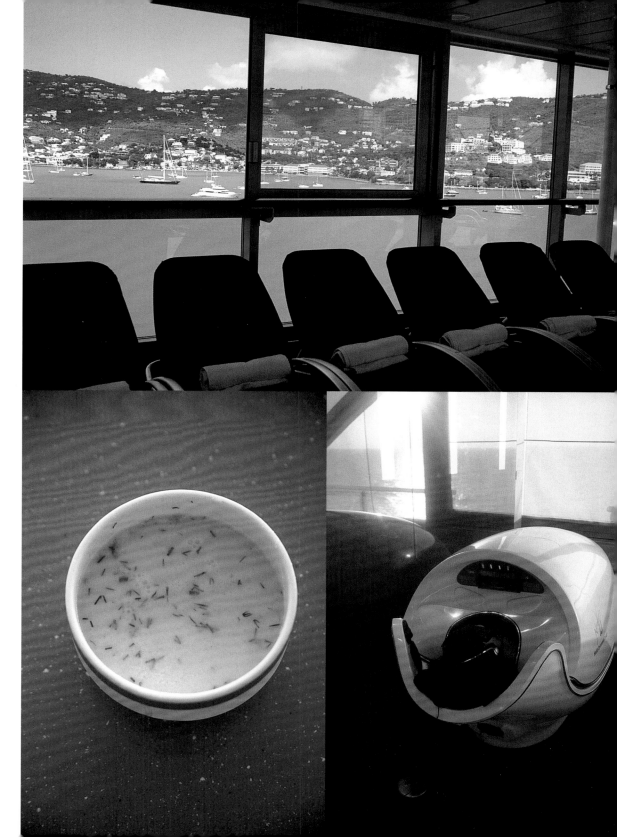

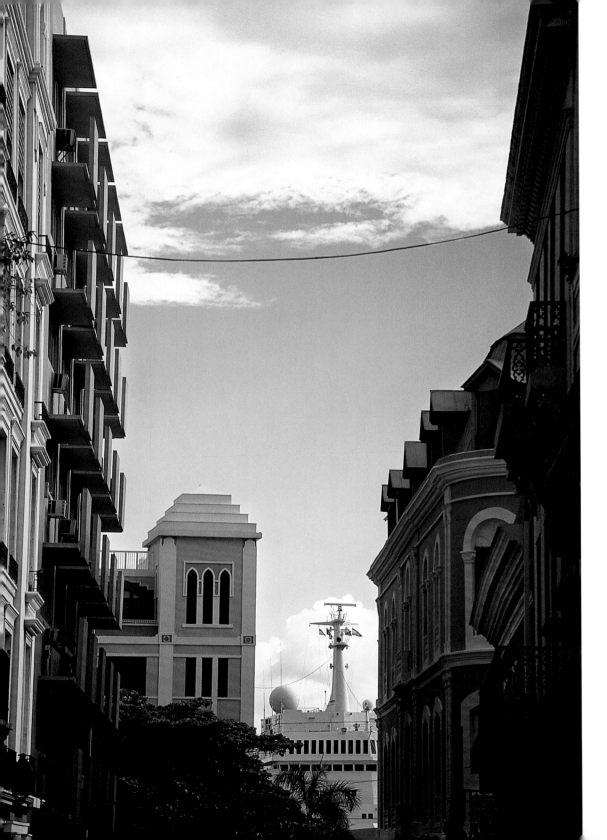

THIS SPA CRUISE IS FOR YOU IF you love cruises as much as you love spas.

THIS SPA CRUISE IS NOT FOR YOU IF you're allergic to crowds or hope to lose weight.

medieval Spanish village—lovely, though not indicative of the country's architecture. In the evening, *Kandela*, a fantastic song and dance show, is performed at an outdoor arena featuring dancers in elaborate, dazzling costumes—instead of Carmen Miranda's fruit-as-headdress, picture giant, green-sequined palm trees—and sexy Latin dance moves that tantalize the eye, dances you probably won't be able to keep up with. (Have you ever seen female dancers flipping men over their backs? You will here.) Other excursions include a hike through the rain forest in Puerto Rico and snorkeling off the island of St. John. (I recommend snorkeling off a small boat. The group I joined at the beach was so large, it frightened away most of the fish.)

St. Thomas is famous for its jewelry deals; there's even a "shopping" class on board that informs you which stores have gems guaranteed by the cruise line. Fighting the hordes of bargain hunters that pour off the pier can be considered a worthy sport for burning off calories. Our last port-of-call, Nassau, in the Bahamas, included a trip to the Atlantis resort on Paradise Island, a frenzied, Vegas-like place. Unfortunately, in recent years, a steep fee of $25 has been added to enter the hotel's main attraction, the aquarium tunnels that cover much of the ground below. You can see more at your local aquarium, so save your money for piña coladas on board.

There are two full days without a port-of-call, the perfect chance to splurge on a "spa ritual," which is a succession of treatments that can include anything from a coconut rub and milk bath to a chakra balancing massage. Whatever you choose, it'll make you float without ever touching the ocean.

PRICE $$–$$$

ROOMS 1,019
Basic, clean & pleasant. Ship's capacity is 1,950 people. If you can afford it and you're even slightly claustrophobic, I recommend a room with a veranda. Some suites have private decks and outdoor hot tubs.

FOOD
Something for everyone—sushi, spa food, appetizers such as salmon and quail eggs, midnight buffets—but a little on the bland side. The food in the main dining room is better than that of the gourmet restaurant for which there is an extra charge.

OUTSTANDING TREATMENTS
Japanese Silk Booster Facial; Coconut Rub and Milk Ritual Wrap; Lonithermie Algae-Detox (electrodes are placed on the body to break-down cellulite).

ACTIVITIES
ONBOARD: Art Auction; Bingo; Shuffleboard.
PORTS-OF-CALL: Hiking; Snorkeling; Horseback Riding; serious Shopping.

CLASSES
Computer; Shopping (where to get best deals at ports-of-call); Aerobics; Pilates; and Yoga.

GETTING THERE
Ship leaves from Port Everglades, Fort Lauderdale, FL

ADDRESS
1050 Caribbean Way
Miami, FL 33132

T 800-529-6918   **F** 800-886-6485   **W** www.celebritycruises.com

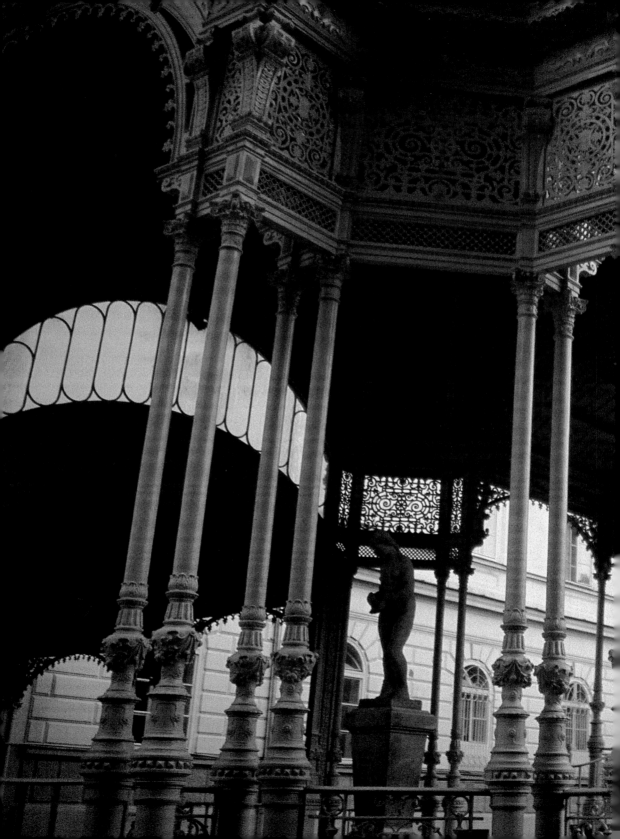

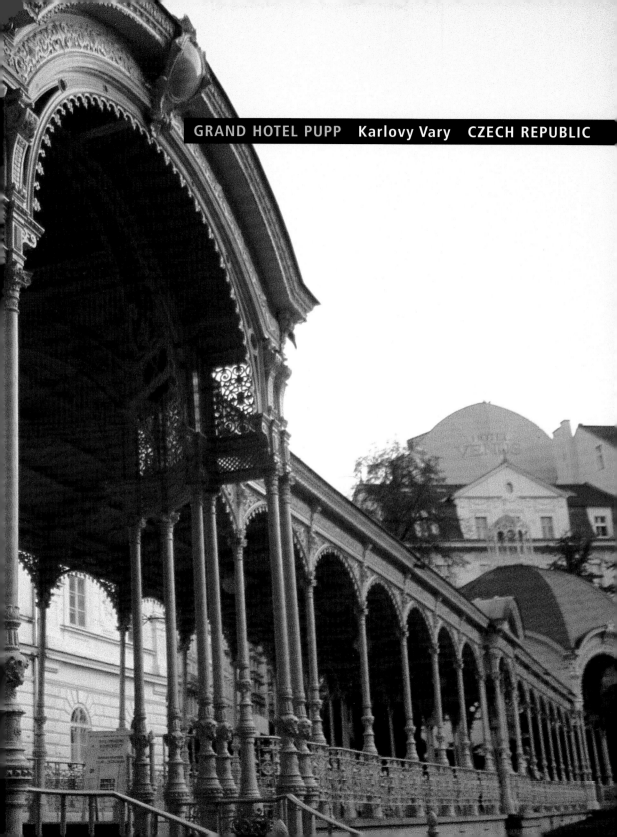

GRAND HOTEL PUPP   Karlovy Vary   CZECH REPUBLIC

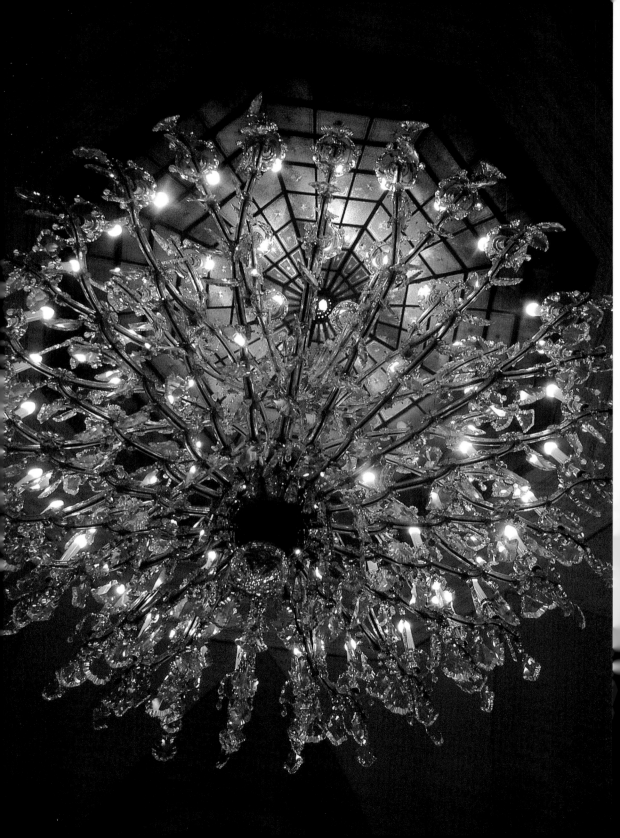

GRAND HOTEL PUPP, KARLOVY VARY, CZECH REPUBLIC

Karlovy Vary is one of those places that seems untouched by time, its daily rituals and rhythms reminiscent of a time centuries past when everything revolved around the waters. In some respects, it is "the mother of all spas."

Surrounded by three mountain ranges, I felt nurtured, as if nothing bad could ever happen here. When so much of a town's history is devoted to health and self-indulgence, a feeling of well-being is bound to permeate the air. Legend has it that the hot springs were discovered in 1350 by Charles the Fourth on a deer hunting expedition when one of the hounds took a dip. The town is named for the king—Karlovy Vary translates as "Charles' spring."

Everything about this ancient spa town encourages visitors to pause and reflect on its charming beauty. Hot springs are sprinkled throughout the town— you can drink from twelve—each with its own healing properties. Some springs are housed in their own gazebo or grand hall; people stroll among them, drinking the waters out of cups with thin porcelain spouts and stopping to look in store windows.

The main street, divided by the Tepla River, winds through the heart of town amid ornate wedding-cake buildings, the Romanesque and rococo architecture somehow managing to appear both imposing and dainty, with grand columned façades and lacy flourishes. Onion-domed churches boldly rise up against the mountains and add to the enchantingly regal aura that makes Karlovy Vary such an intriguing sight to behold.

If visitors aren't drinking from the springs, they're patronizing one of the cafes, having a coffee dolloped with whipped cream, and perhaps a pastry. Like Vienna, Karlovy Vary is known for its confectionary, and there seems to be no guilt in indulging one's sweet tooth in-between taking the waters.

The Hotel Pupp's spa doctor, Milada Sarova, will recommend a regimen using water from different springs, depending on what ails you. Tests of the water show it to contain minerals vital to a healthy body, improving digestion, boosting the immune system, and reducing inflammation. A prescription is required before soaking in the mineral waters at the town spa. "Some of these waters can cause blood pressure to rise," she says. "We need to know what we're dealing with."

Dr. Sarova's office is next to the Hotel Pupp, which was built in 1701 by Georg Johann Pupp, a renowned pastry chef. Karlovy Vary, once known as Karlsbad, hosted an endless stream of luminaries in the nineteenth century, when it was a summer playground for Goethe, Mozart, and other artists, politicians, and royals.

Amid the grandeur and elegance, a spiritual presence pervades the valley. On top of the mountain, behind the hotel, is a cross with Jesus looking down. And in the center of town is a synagogue decorated with a glimmering gold star—an important monument in a village that made Hitler an honorary citizen during the Nazi occupation.

To get to the main spa in town—called the Castle—you must walk a few steps up a hill near the synagogue. It is worth the climb. Once inside, the place is all soothing pastels and marble. Rock walls are ballast to the celestial atmosphere.

The main pool, filled with mineral water and surrounded by windows overlooking the street, lets in just the right amount of natural light. Every few hours, the shades are drawn and a light and music show ensues, complete with shapes of mythic gods beamed onto the carved granite walls. Like many such shows, once the novelty wears off it can get tiring, but it doesn't detract from the overall splendid atmosphere.

After one afternoon in this mineral pool followed by a carbonated bath and a hot-cold Kneipp water-path treatment, you may find yourself feeling as if you've just had a couple glasses of bubbly—light, happy, and a little tipsy, as if nothing could ever bother you again. For you've been nurtured by the mother of all spas.

THIS SPA IS FOR YOU IF you're interested in taking an old-fashioned "water cure" in a luxurious setting.

THIS SPA IS NOT FOR YOU IF spa food is very important to you.

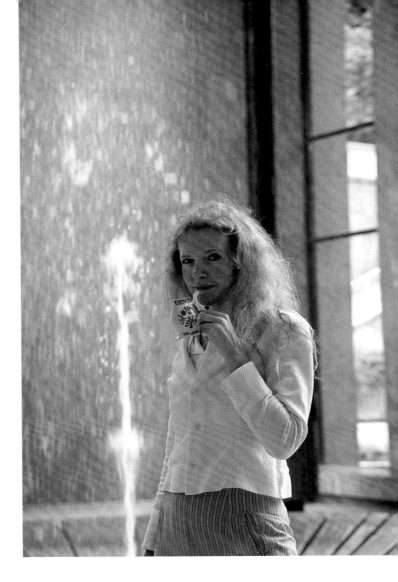

PRICE $$–$$$

ROOMS 199
Some are elegantly appointed and others are sumptuous and luxurious.

FOOD
The hotel's main restaurant serves Czech and international cuisine.

Czech food is hearty and carb-heavy (dumplings made with white flour and gravy are a favorite). For low-fat choices, the restaurant offers decent salmon and sole. **CAFÉ ELEFANT** down the block is legendary for its pastry confections.

OUTSTANDING TREATMENTS
The Carbonated Bath at the Castle, the town's main spa.

ACTIVITIES
Walking wooded paths; Hiking; Horseback Riding; Tennis; Squash; and Golf.

GETTING THERE
A 90-minute drive from Prague. 2 hours by train or bus.

ADDRESS
Mirove namesti 2
360-91 Karlovy Vary,
Czech Republic

T 420-353-109-111   **F** 420-353-224-032   **E** main@pupp.kpgroup.cz   **W** www.pupp.cz

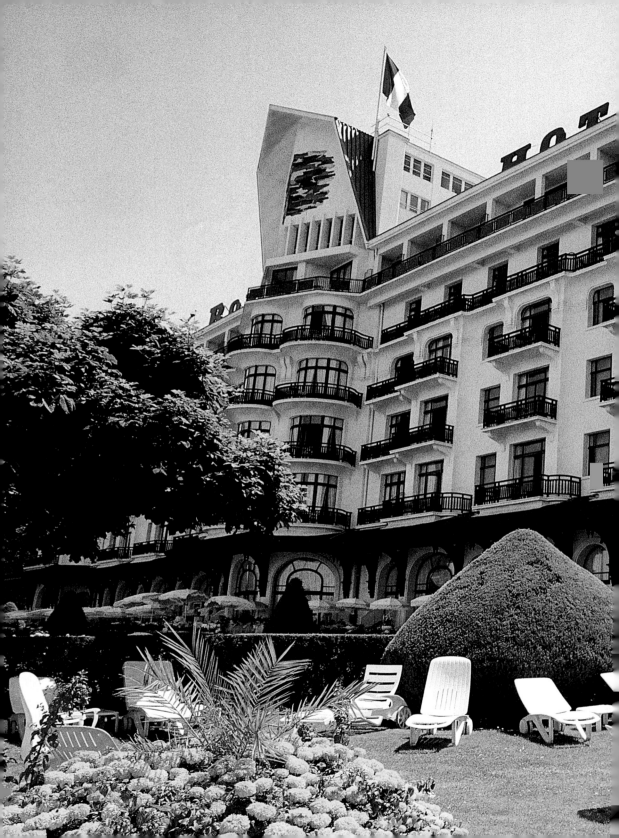

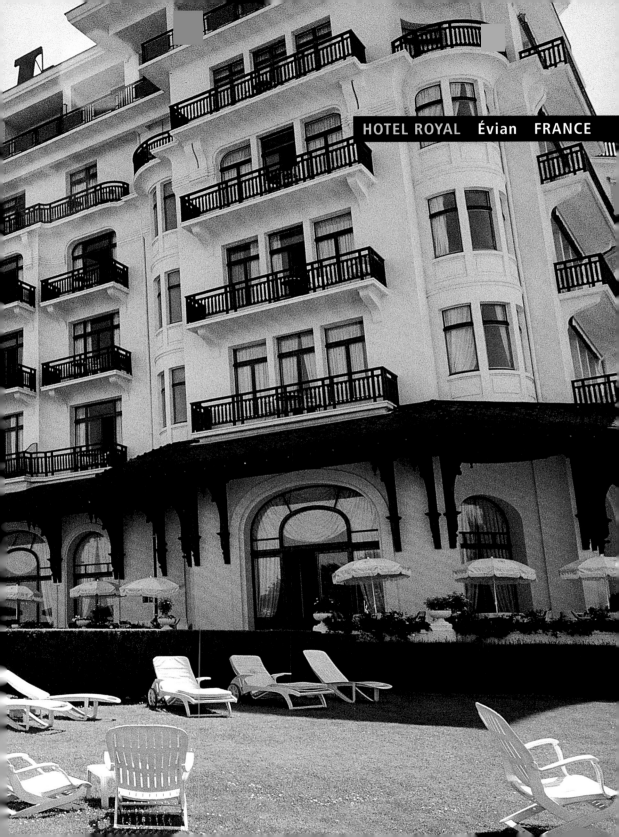

HOTEL ROYAL Évian FRANCE

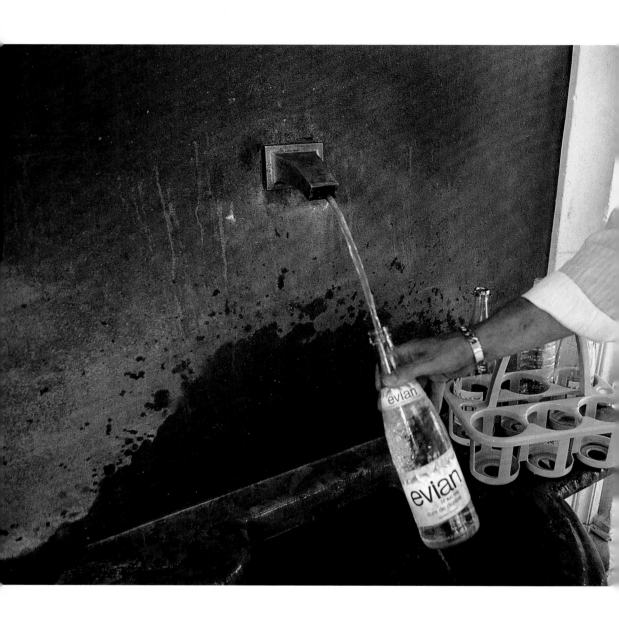

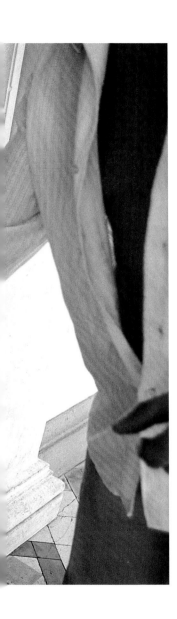

HOTEL ROYAL, ÉVIAN, FRANCE

The Hotel Royal is a world of crystal chandeliers, plush carpets, and sumptuous blue draperies that swirl like evening gowns on a ballroom floor. From the rolling acres of velvety green, perfectly manicured lawn to the blue, syrup-smooth surface of Lake Geneva (which matches the drapes), everything about the Hotel Royal is, well, royal. Set in the foothills of the snow-capped Alps, the hotel was built during the late nineteenth-century Belle Epoque—the golden age of French art and culture—in honor of England's King Edward the Seventh. The hotel is part of the Royal Parc Évian, forty-two acres of glorious gardens on which also sits the more casual Hotel Hermitage.

The Hotel Royal may seem a bit stuffy at first: Painted dome ceilings and delicate French furniture always make me feel underdressed (especially if I'm wearing the rumpled black jacket I couldn't fit into my suitcase). But the pleasant surprise here is the air of casual bonhomie that continually peeks out from behind the drapes and bounces from the chandeliers. To many Americans, the scariest thing about France is the French. And if you have ever been growled at by Parisian waiters, the attitude at the Hotel Royal will seem quite revolutionary: The staff, though indubitably French, is polite, cheerful, and positively gracious.

Of course, they still insist on calling Lake Geneva "Lake Leman" (they simply can't bear to call it by the same name as the Swiss), but they are devoted to making guests feel royally comfortable. Need an electric adapter for your American blow dryer? No problem: someone will be up within five minutes. Need a new robe delivered? There in five minutes. And your glass of Evian never empties; someone is always there to top it off. The source of this world-famous mineral water is less than a mile away.

Guests are made to feel they have the run of this royal residence. A private elevator leads to the spa from each floor, so you can wear a fluffy robe without having to walk through the lobby. The spa itself is all Asian elegance with orchids and the clean lines of polished wood. A standout treatment is called Korean Relaxation, which is similar to a Thai massage, but more gentle. My therapist, a Russian woman who had lived in France for ten years, kept telling me, "Pretend you are dead, let me do ze work." I thought I had been doing a good job of that, but she admonished me that it was not good enough. "You keep anticipating what I'm going to do and you try to help me," she explained. Earlier that day, she had massaged the president of Cameroon and he had just "let go," she said. "But Americans have a hard time doing this."

Unlike in other thermal spas, bathing in the waters is not popular. The only swimming pool filled with Evian is at a spa in town. Évian does have its own ancient legend of a miraculous healing. A poor shepherd, it is told, wished to marry a wealthy man's daughter. When the father grew sick, the shepherd urged him to drink the water. The father was

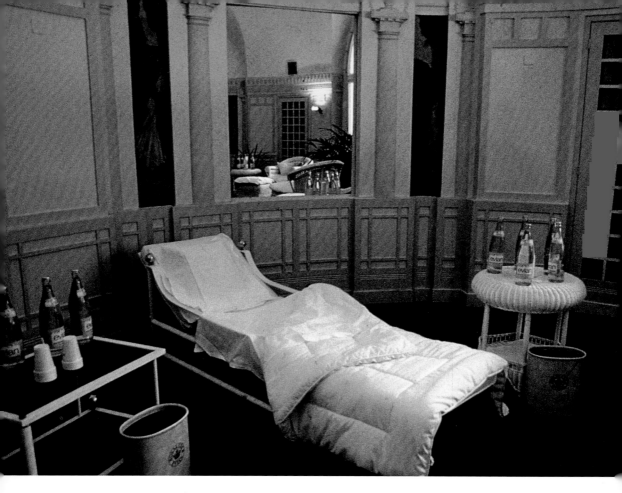

PRICE $$$

ROOMS 154
Elegantly appointed, offering spectacular views of either Lake Geneva or the gardens.

FOOD
A low-fat gourmet restaurant serves French Zen spa food (herb-spiced cod on a bed of lentils, and for dessert, apples in an egg and cream zabaglione sauce). Be forewarned: lunch for two can run up to $100. **LA VERANDA** offers a can't-miss buffet lunch with several varieties of cheese, salads, fish, soups, and bread.

You could skip the entrée (free-range meats from the local market) to save room for dessert (all the crème brûlée and chocolate tortes you can eat). A high-end French dining room includes impeccable cuisine and service.

OUTSTANDING TREATMENTS
Rasul Mud Treatment, a fancy steam bath (derived from ancient Egypt) with decorative tiles and twinkling lights on the ceiling—said to enhance absorption of mud and lotions; Korean Relaxation (see main text for description).

ACTIVITIES
Horseback Riding; Golf; Helicopter Rides; Hot-Air Ballooning over Mont-Blanc; Sailing and Canoeing on Lake Geneva; Dogsledding; Alpine Skiing; Gambling at Évian Casino.

CLASSES
Aerobics (in English and French).

NEARBY ATTRACTIONS
Ferry ride across Lake Geneva to the lovely Swiss town of Lausanne.

FOR CHILDREN
A children's club for ages 2–11 offers indoor and

outdoor play areas, workshops, a dance studio, theater, and multimedia room. Open daily from 9 A.M. to 6 P.M. There's also a club for teenagers that includes sports and daily excursions.

GETTING THERE
A 45-minute drive from Geneva airport.

ADDRESS
South Bank of Lake Geneva 74501 Évian-Les-Bains France

T 33-4-50-26-85-00   **F** 33-4-50-75-61-00   **E** reservation@royalparcevian.com   **W** www.royalparcevian.com

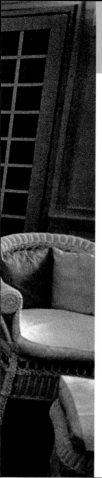

cured, and the shepherd was able to marry his love. But no one today takes the healing properties very seriously. "We try to de-emphasize the medicinal aspect of the waters," said Alain Spieser, Hotel Royal's marketing director. "We want to focus on this as a place to de-stress."

Évian's town spa also offers a swimming program for new parents and their babies. Studies show that babies who are exposed to water at an early age are less fearful of it when they are older. If nothing else, swimming is a relaxing, fun way to bond with your baby. The one-week program begins with an introductory class in which parents hold their infants in the water; in later classes, the babies float in plastic boats. Finally, if they're ready, they are dunked underwater. This is not as alarming as it sounds. Under the age of nine months, babies haven't developed the automatic gag reflex, so they are able to remain briefly underwater without discomfort or danger.

The Hotel Royal welcomes children, and has a children's club supervised by pediatric nurses. Tykes roam about with their sippy-cups full of Evian water, like little royals.

By the time I checked out, I felt quite regal myself, rumpled black jacket notwithstanding. And just a little closer to learning to "let go."

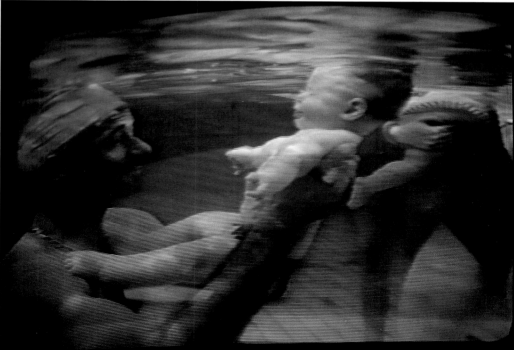

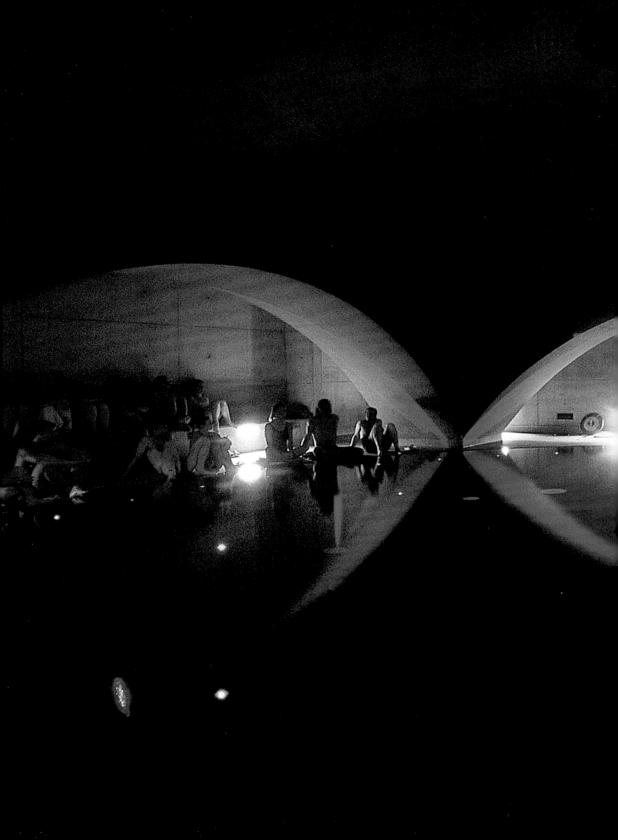

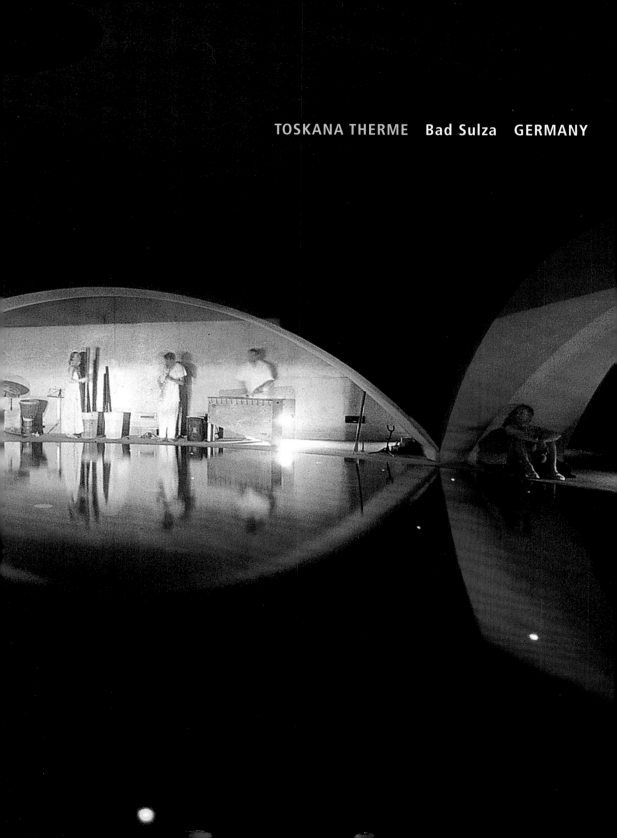

TOSKANA THERME   Bad Sulza   GERMANY

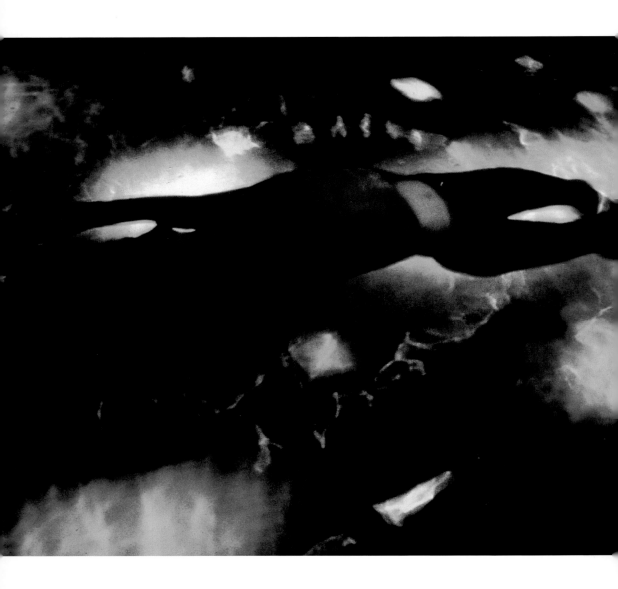

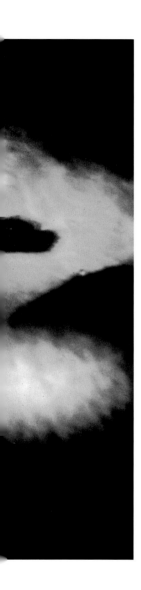

TOSKANA THERME, BAD SULZA, GERMANY

The main attraction of Toskana Therme is the sublime concept called Liquid Sound, a marriage of music and water, with a touch of light thrown in. Pools of saltwater featuring a built-in, state-of-the-art sound system are housed in a futuristic, domed building with floor-to-ceiling windows, through which is seen a landscape often called "the Tuscany of Eastern Europe."

Not many spas have pools with underwater music, and the ones that do don't offer a light show to go with it. Toskana Therme ("Toskana" refers to the Tuscan scenery, "Therme" to its thermal springs) is the Carnegie Hall of water relaxation; it's what every spa with music and water therapy should aspire to be. In recent years, studies have shown that listening to music can lower blood pressure and improve immune system function. The water comes from an underground saltwater reservoir that is so dense that you quickly spring to the surface like a buoy. At first, floating on my back, I was a bit squeamish about getting water in my ears (though pool policy requires bathing caps, water found its way in). But in my quest to follow the advice of massage therapists everywhere I told myself to "let go" and "surrender to the experience."

Except for the sound of lapping water, I was alone with my thoughts, feeling suspended in time and weightless, as I merged with the water into liquid sound. Looking up at the domed ceiling, I watched iridescent pinks and blues dissolve into the ether and return as different shapes. Closing my eyes, I relaxed to the reverberations of the violin and cello, and let the music massage me, lulling me further into myself.

Liquid Sound sprang from the creative mind of artist and musician Micky Remann during a research expedition to study orca whales in the Canadian Pacific. "It was like listening to a beautiful otherworldly symphony, and very relaxing—almost trance-like," he says. "I thought: *What else could have that effect?*" Remann compiled hundreds of combinations of music, mostly classical and sounds from nature, which extend through the water in relaxing waves. But the selections can be quite varied. You may hear jazz, tango, and, of course, the New Age Elvis of spa music, Enya.

"Music sounds different in the water—you experience it more fully," says Remann. This is partly because sound travels faster through water. And because 70 percent of the human body is composed of water, it's no surprise that Liquid Sound will have you feeling the music in every pore.

The appeal of Liquid Sound has spread to Berlin, where Toskana Therme has a sister spa called Liquidrom (pictured in the introduction to this review). "Many people come in on their lunch hour or after work when they need to unwind or find inspiration," says Remann. "Creative people, like artists and writers, say it helps them when they're blocked."

The experience is further heightened during "underwater" concerts, which both spas sponsor at least

THIS SPA IS FOR YOU IF you're interested in German culture and history and you love water and music.

THIS SPA IS NOT FOR YOU IF you prefer your spa travel completely luxurious.

once a month. Live orchestras perform everything from Handel's Water Music to the works of Liszt and Bach, and the audience absorbs it all while floating. Underwater ballet is also performed.

It is fitting that spa owners Marion Schneider and Klaus Boehm plan to turn the former East German spa town of Bad Sulza into a cultural mecca. Just a twenty-minute train ride away is the city of Weimar, at one time an intellectual and arts center and home to many renowned composers and artists, including Goethe, Wagner, and Bach.

Today, you can feel the ghosts of the greats as you walk along the cobblestone streets of this historic town. Unlike most towns in this part of Germany, much of the architecture survived after the bombing of World War II. And since the fall of the Berlin Wall, it's been spruced up. Today it virtually shimmers with life. Bright greens, yellows, and pinks, with ornamental flourishes of gold, adorn the buildings as they wind their way towards the *Marktplatz*.

Sit in a cafe near Goethe's house, and listen to the gentle trickle of water from the nearby fountain. At times, you can even hear a violin, the notes floating through a window from the nearby conservatory. Water and music, joined together once again.

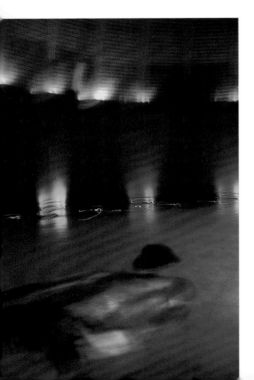

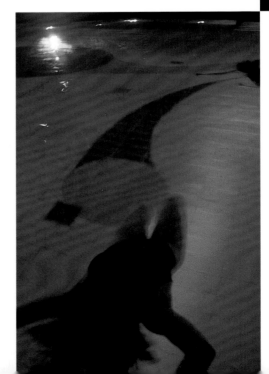

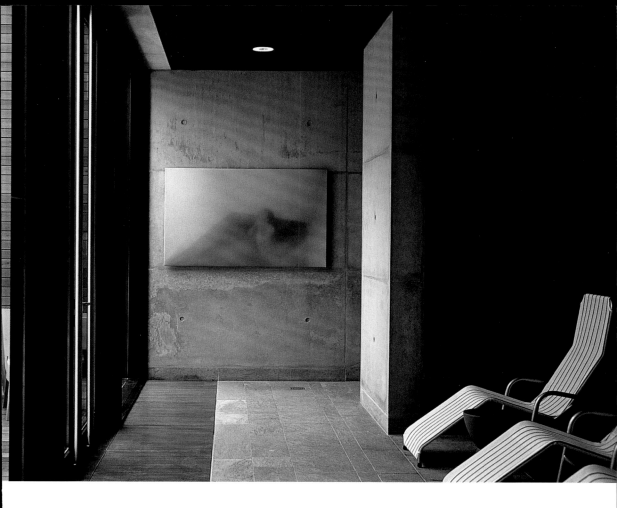

PRICE $

ROOMS 81
Basic, clean & pleasant.

FOOD
The main restaurant in the hotel serves a buffet breakfast of cheese, bread, and cereals. Lunch and dinner, also buffet, offer a healthy, fresh selection of soups, lean meats, and vegetarian entrées. A cafe near the pools serves pizza and pasta.

OUTSTANDING TREATMENTS
Like many European spas, this one has a medical clinic on-site (primarily treating skin ailments, such as psoriasis, with saltwater pools and light boxes). It also offers colonics, acupuncture, and osteopathic manipulation. As for spa services, try the Milk Bath or the Ayurvedic Herbal Massage. At the pools, Aqua Wellness treatments are offered (similar to *Watsu*, or floating water massage).

CLASSES
Aqua-Aerobics; Pilates; and Yoga (all in German).

NEARBY ATTRACTIONS
Weimar (check out Goethe's houses and Liszt's home), Leipzig, Dresden.

GETTING THERE
A 3-hour drive from Frankfurt, and an hour's drive from Leipzig airport.

ADDRESS
Wunderwaldstrasse 2
99518 Bad Sulza
Germany

T 49-36461-92881   **F** 49-36461-92095   **E** info@toskana-therme.de   **W** www.toskana-therme.de

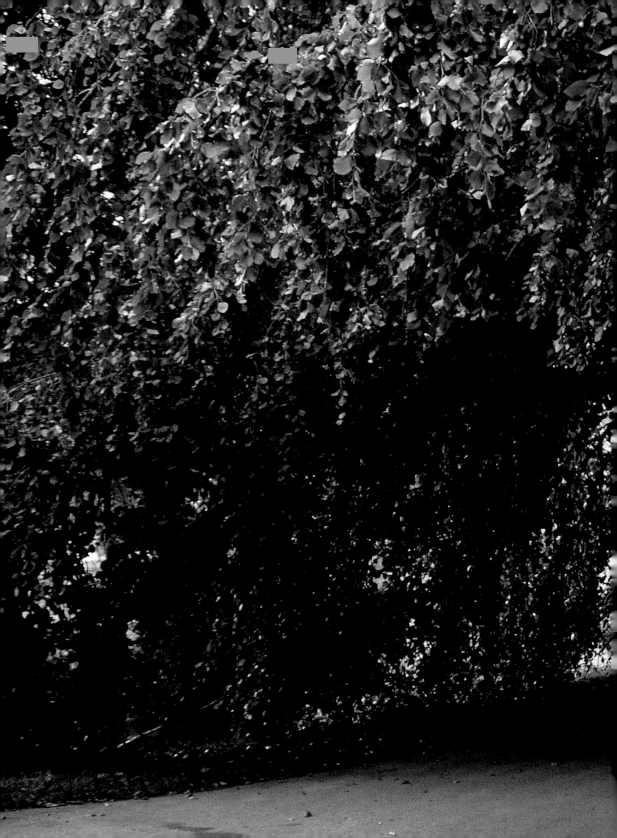

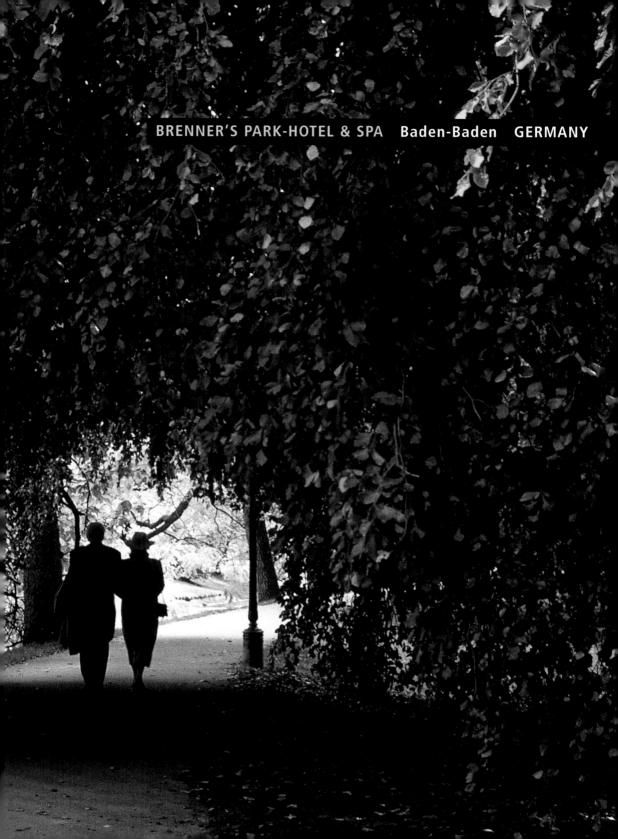

BRENNER'S PARK-HOTEL & SPA   Baden-Baden   GERMANY

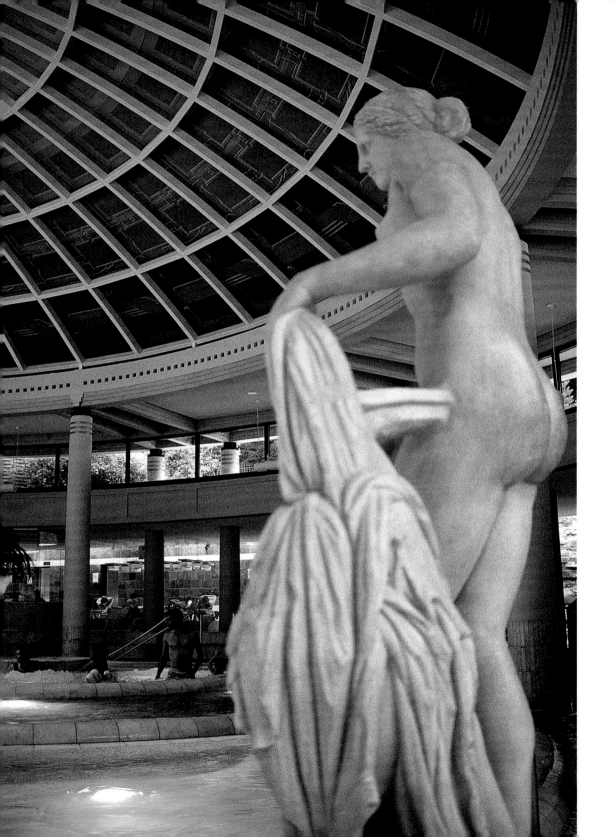

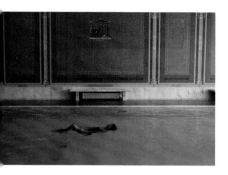

BRENNER'S PARK-HOTEL & SPA, BADEN-BADEN, GERMANY

Fountains are everywhere in Baden-Baden. Water gods strut and sea nymphs dance among them, and the sprays of water sing as if from the score of a trickling, splashing symphony. Perhaps this is one reason that, historically, the town has always attracted so many musicians. Brahms was so taken with it that he built a villa he called his "composing cavern." Franz Liszt also composed much of his most memorable music here.

Baden-Baden is rich in history, and in addition to the great composers, its devotees are numerous. Roman soldiers by the thousands bathed in its hot springs for sustenance before and after battle. Roman Emperor Caracalla, the Donald Trump of his day, ordered the stonework of the town bathhouse upgraded with marble and granite. And like the Donald, he named it after himself: Caracalla Thermae.

By the nineteenth century, Baden-Baden was established as the summer capital of Europe, attracting scores of great artists and writers, such as Delacroix, Stendhal, and Balzac, as well as royalty, including Queen Victoria, Napoleon the Third, and Edward the Seventh. Some came to cure what ailed them, but many came for the scenic beauty of the Black Forest, and the clear air of the Oos Valley. Others came for the gambling at what was once one of the most famous casinos in the world. Today, the casino is still a big draw, and has maintained its nineteenth-century neo-baroque splendor, with a display of impressive oil paintings on the walls and glistening chandeliers that shine from the ceiling.

The Germans are very serious about thermal waters— a spa visit is covered by medical insurance. And Baden-Baden is the most famous spa town in a nation that treasures its spas. The word *bad* is German for bath; it has been said that Baden-Baden was so named because the baths were so superior they had to be acknowledged twice.

Next door to the casino is the Pump Room (Trinkhalle), where Germans suffering liver ailments and digestive problems come to drink the waters. Across town, Emperor Caracalla still has a bathhouse named after him, a modern rendition of steel and glass built on top of the ruins of a Roman campsite, which can still be seen beneath the building. At the Caracalla-Therme, you can enjoy both indoor and outdoor thermal pools, as well as various water treatments, such as neck showers and whirlpools.

The town's older bathhouse, Friedrichsbad, dates from 1877 and has hardly changed since Brahms came for a soak. You can alternate between a dip in a hot plunge pool and a cold one in a beautiful setting of domed ceilings, decorative tiles, and Corinthian columns. But Americans be forewarned: the Germans do much of their public bathing in the nude. Be prepared to see many a droopy butt, and everything else besides. Older men seem particularly

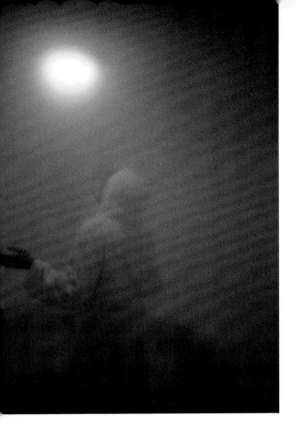
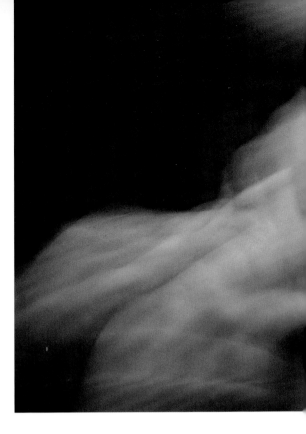

PRICE $$$$

ROOMS 100
Elegantly appointed.

FOOD
Three restaurants, one very formal, requiring jackets and ties for dinner; a more casual dining room; and a breakfast spot. Spa cuisine is prepared on request.

OUTSTANDING TREATMENTS
Milk-Honey Body Mask; Four-Hands Massage; and Meridian-Acupressure Massage.

ACTIVITIES
Bathing in a historic bathhouse (Friedrichsbad); Strolling through Old Town; Concerts at Festival Hall and the neoclassical Kurhaus; Horseback Riding; Golf; Tennis; and Hiking.

CLASSES
Water Fitness; Pilates; and Yoga (all in German and English).

NEARBY ATTRACTIONS
Medieval Lichtenthal Cloister; the Black Forest; the wine country of Rebland; the towns of Heidelberg and Strasbourg.

GETTING THERE
2 hours by car and train from Frankfurt airport.

ADDRESS
Schillerstrasse 4-6
76530 Baden-Baden
Germany

T 49-7221-9000   **F** 49-7221-38772   **E** info@brenners.com   **W** www.brenners.com

THIS SPA IS FOR YOU IF you want romance and luxury in an old-world spa town.
THIS SPA IS NOT FOR YOU IF you want to follow a serious exercise regimen and strict low-fat diet.

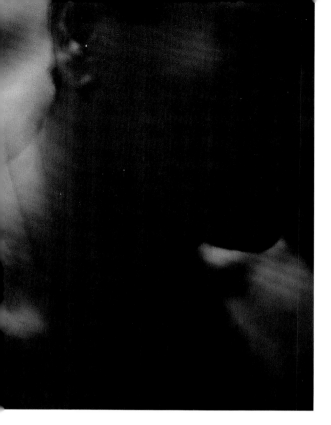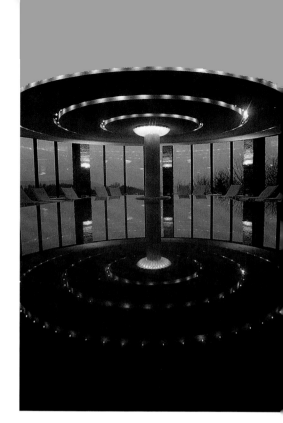

immodest, padding around frog-like without a care in the world. A more pleasant sight is the flocks of nubile girls from Japan, another hot-springs-loving culture.

If you're craving privacy, you can always try the spa at Brenner's Park-Hotel, a celebrated fixture of old-world elegance. In the lobby, you may also experience some old-world stuffiness, but once inside the spa, the atmosphere is spare and relaxed. As with many recently renovated spas, it has an Asian theme, including a Japanese garden and jasmine-scented steam room. There is also a special suite available for private parties of up to four, offering such amenities as a marble whirlpool bath, the services of a butler, and a sauna featuring heated quartzite benches to prepare and relax you for the maximum benefits of a massage.

At night, Baden-Baden is still an inspiration for artists, and just about everyone else. The town is very much a cultural center, with many music festivals, concerts, theater performances and gallery openings to choose from. As you walk the cobblestone streets, past well-scrubbed ancient buildings, flower boxes, and iron lattice-work balconies, you may even hear a Brahms concerto bubbling up from the fountains. The music may be coming from an adjacent concert hall, or it may just be in your mind.

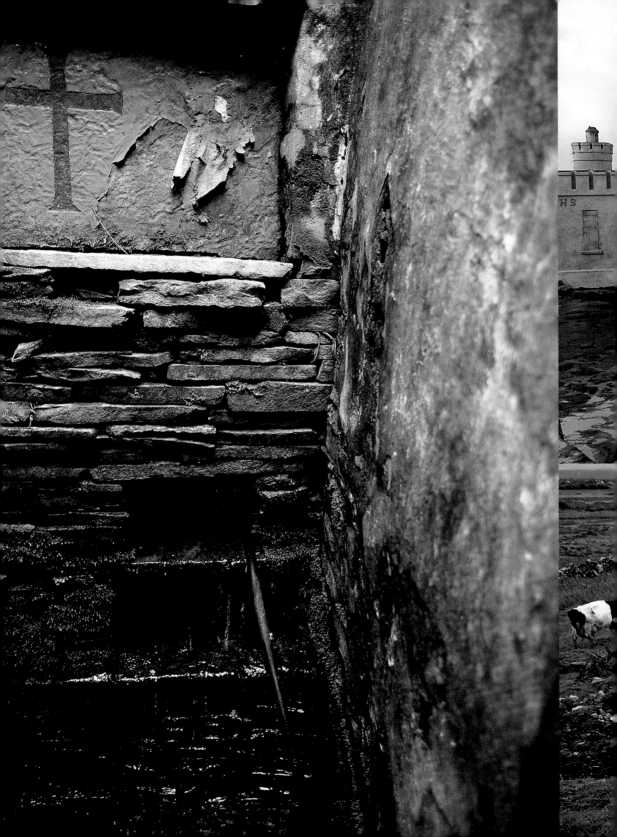

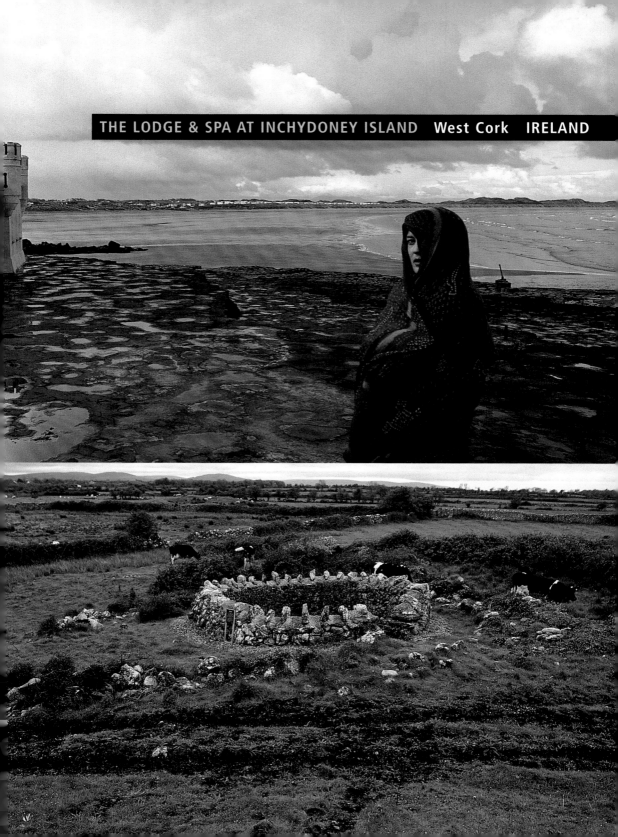

THIS SPA IS FOR YOU IF you love the ocean and the Irish.

THIS SPA IS NOT FOR YOU IF you prefer tropical beaches.

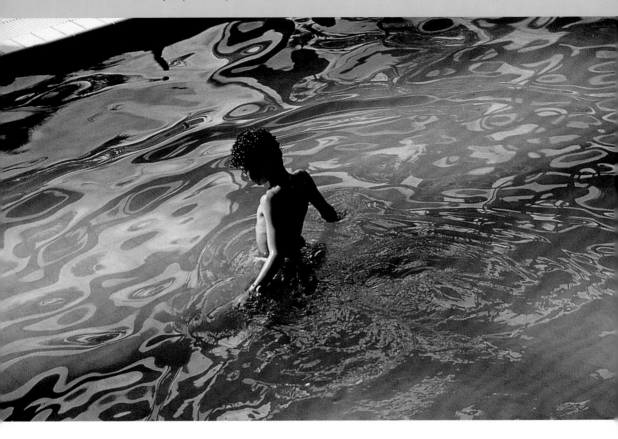

PRICE $$–$$$

ROOMS 63
Basic, clean & pleasant. All rooms have ocean views, but if you're in the mood for splurging, the three suites have breathtaking views of the water, making you feel like you're suspended above it.

FOOD
The main restaurant offers creative healthy fare, using organic produce and vegetables. Some are low-fat, such as feta pockets with spinach, and others are rich, including every kind of salmon you can imagine—moussed, sliced, poached, or grilled. A more traditional pub-restaurant is on the ground floor.

OUTSTANDING TREATMENTS
Algotherapy (algae mud and a wrap).

ACTIVITIES
Horseback Riding; Biking; Clay-Pigeon Shooting; Off-Road Driving; and Walking (through the dunes). Golf and Deep-Sea Fishing nearby.

CLASSES
Aqua Fitness; Chi Kung; Tai Chi; and Yoga.

NEARBY ATTRACTIONS
The charming town of Clonakilty, full of pubs, shops, and nightlife.

It's also the place where Michael Collins (Ireland's George Washington) lived as a youth. His home and a memorial are right in town.

GETTING THERE
A 45-minute drive from the Cork airport.

ADDRESS
Clonakilty
West Cork, Ireland

T 353-23-33143   **F** 353-23-35229   **E** reservations@inchydoneyisland.com   **W** www.inchydoneyisland.com

THE LODGE & SPA AT INCHYDONEY ISLAND, WEST CORK, IRELAND

Like so much of the Irish countryside, Inchydoney Island evokes a mystical, end-of-the-world peace. The majority of visitors associate Ireland with its green lushness, not realizing that it also has a rich history of water worship going back thousands of years. Wells devoted to the saints still dot the land, their waters long believed to cure blindness, infertility, and other maladies. St. Brigid, particularly beloved by the Irish, has many wells devoted to her. In the town of Faughart, pilgrims tear off bits of their clothing and hang them over an ancient well, each torn piece symbolizing an affliction that they hope she will heal.

The spa at Inchydoney Island offers more modern hydrotherapies. After distinguished careers spent developing several successful resorts in the Caribbean, Michael and Hazel Johnston wanted to build a place of their own. They searched the world for the perfect beach and found it in the south of Ireland, home of revolutionary hero Michael Collins, Murphy's stout, and plenty of friendly pubs.

The Johnstons chose wisely. No palm trees or balmy breezes grace Inchydoney Island, but its timeless beauty rivals any Caribbean reef. The presence of the sea pervades the Lodge, where rooms, the main restaurant, and the indoor pool all have a view. The beach is at its most romantic when there is a slight chill in the air. The gentle wash of breaking waves lulls you to sleep and greets you in the morning. And the invigorating scent of sea air is everywhere, filling your lungs with pure enchanting energy. Afterwards, warm up with a sherry by the fire while a pianist plays Irish airs.

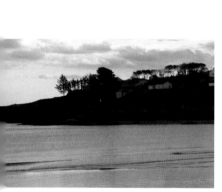

The resort claims to be Ireland's only true thalasso-therapy spa. *Thalassa*, Greek for "sea water," is touted by many European doctors for treatment of sore joints, headaches, and many other stress-related ailments. At Inchydoney, seawater is pumped daily into the pool, and bathers can relax in a host of whirlpools, showers, and fountains. "Unless the seawater is refreshed each day, nutrients die," says Dr. Christian Jost, who designed the thalasso pool here as well as numerous others in France. Inchydoney's thalasso pool is no deeper than four and a half feet so even non-swimmers can use it. It's a little like taking a series of water rides: There's a pulsing shoulder massage at one station, and at another, "bubble seats" that give a gentle champagne-like tickling upon the backs of your thighs (or bottom).

The town of Clonakilty, a short taxi ride away, is an archetypal Irish village with a surprisingly lively nightlife. The pubs fairly burst with music to suit every taste. Most visitors will doubtless opt for one of the folk pubs, where musicians sit in a circle and play the traditional jigs and reels of Ireland. As you tap your toes, and maybe even kick up your heels a bit, you might want to sample another of Ireland's famed liquid cures: a tall, dark pint of stout.

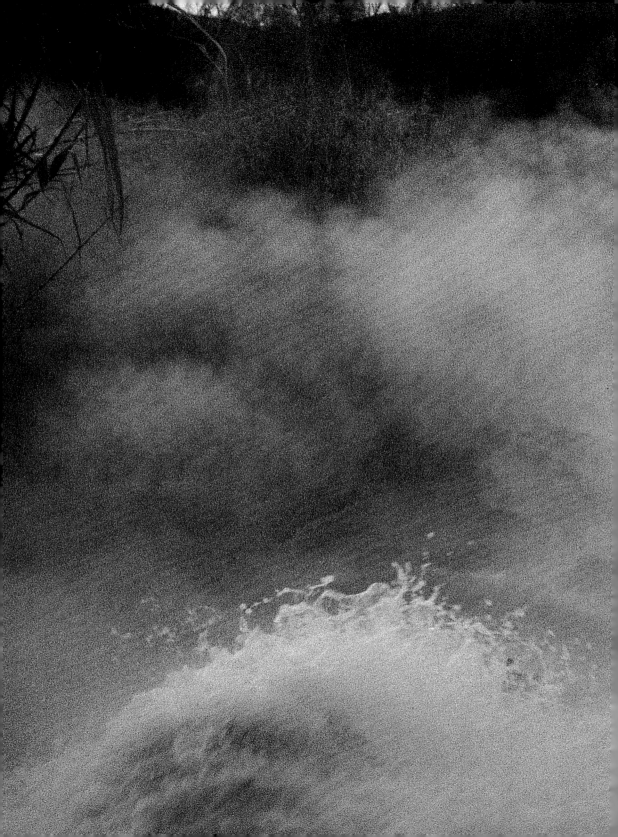

TERME DI SATURNIA   Tuscany   ITALY

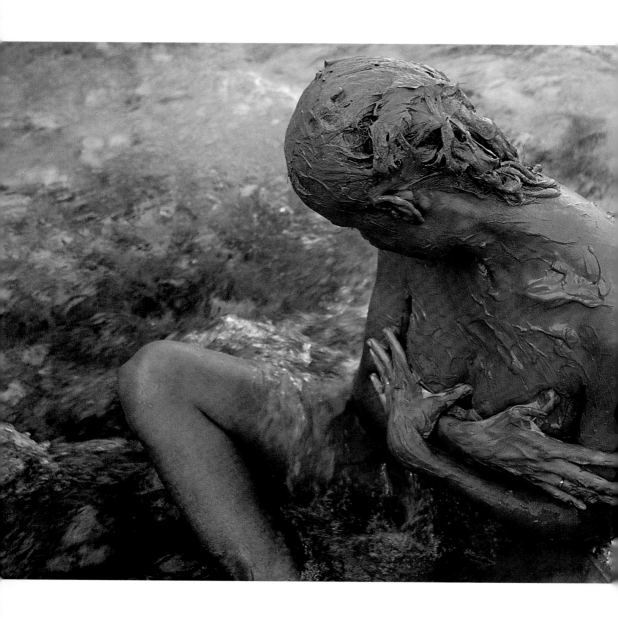

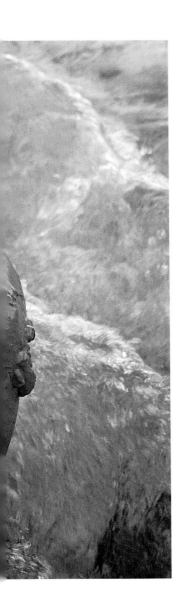

TERME DI SATURNIA, TUSCANY, ITALY

There are times when the lounge resembles a Fellini movie.
A woman in a white fuzzy robe, black sunglasses, and a leopard-
print headband tilts her head toward the ceiling, and blows
smoke rings. She has just emerged from the pool, but she
wears lipstick as red as a fire truck. Her friend, in burgundy
leather trousers, lights up as well. A distinguished-looking
gentleman downs a cup of high-octane espresso as he reads
the paper. At another table, a waiter delivers three glasses of
red wine and one low-fat raspberry smoothie. And through
the window, a plume of moody steam rises off the pool, which
resembles an enchanted cauldron in a fairy tale.

This vision comes from thermal springs bubbling up
at a rate of 160 gallons per second. The 98-degree pool is
the central attraction of this spa resort, which dates back to
the time of the Etruscans. The water runs through volcanic
soil that saturates it with just the right combination of
sulfur and bicarbonate to make you swoon. One fifteen-
minute soak can be an intoxicating experience, like drinking
just enough champagne.

The Romans named the site "Saturnia" for Saturn, the
patron god of Rome, and built the Via Clodia, a road leading
here from the city still traveled today. According to legend,
Saturn became so enraged by the constant fighting among
mortal men that he threw a lightning bolt to earth and struck
a volcano. Hot sulfurous water was brought forth, embracing
the land and calming the people.

This is easier to believe once you've spent time in these
serene pastel blue waters. Their warmth embraces you
indeed, and you soon forget their sulfurous smell and
surrender to a euphoric rush that makes the world appear a
better place. I couldn't get enough. My first day started
with a multi-jet treatment, a sort of whirlpool mineral bath.
Next on the agenda was an aqua-aerobics class in the small
mineral pool; both activities conducted in Italian (except for
the words "Elvis the pelvis," accompanied by a whirling of
hips, which the Italians responded to with gales of laughter).
I visited the terraced waterfalls in the afternoon, which are
a five-minute walk from the spa. I luxuriated in those waters
and continued to feel wonderful until I got back to my room.
I then experienced a dull, throbbing headache, not unlike
a hangover. All of those minerals can go to your head. The spa
advises newcomers to limit their time in the water to about
twenty minutes the first few days.

The hangover was quickly remedied by a pasta dinner
with, believe it or not, pumpkin, mussels, garlic, and olive oil.
The Tuscans do amazing things with pasta, and it was always
melt-in-your-mouth fresh here. The menu plan is best
described as moderate hedonism—typical hearty fare of the
region, such as roasted rabbit and risotto with beef filet and
red wine, cooked with less fattening oils and slightly smaller
portions. And, of course, this being Italy, an impressive
selection of wine is served with both lunch and dinner.

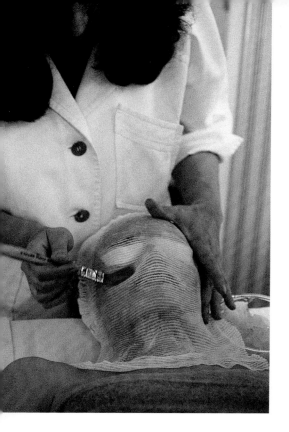

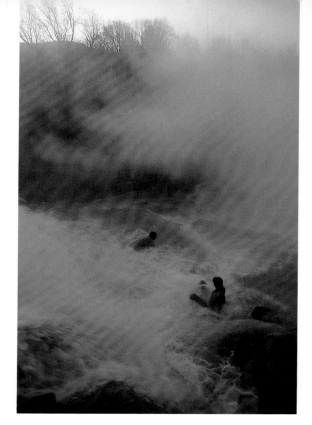

For exercise, you may enjoy walking the medieval hill towns nearby, in lieu of going to the gym. Throughout Tuscany, these towns rise like jeweled kingdoms amid the rolling countryside of ancient stone terraces, wheat fields, and vineyards. Pitigliano beckons visitors from a distance as it is built on *tufa*, a soft, malleable, but sturdy rock. High on its hill, weathered brick buildings emanate fortitude from across the centuries.

You'll wander the winding cobblestone streets like a child in a maze, fascinated at every turn: an Etruscan cave here, a charming, leaning old house there, and spectacular views of the muted green cypress trees of the valley below. An outdoor cafe is never far off. One glass of wine won't hurt. Step into Fellini's imagination and enjoy *La Dolce Vita*.

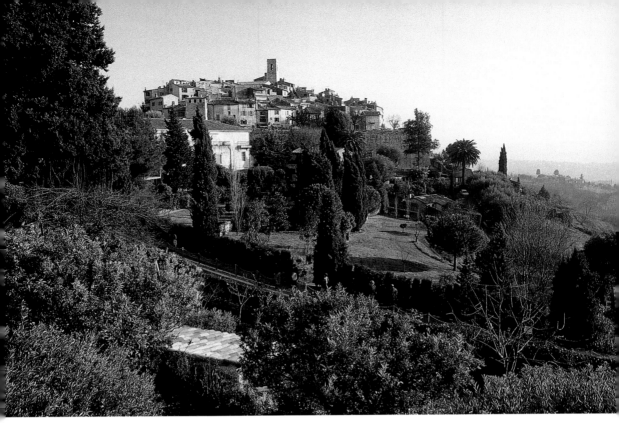

PRICE $$

ROOMS 90
Elegantly appointed.

FOOD
The main restaurant serves all meals. Breakfast buffet; superb antipasto buffet accompanies lunch and dinner. There is no "spa food" here, but plenty of fresh, healthy Mediterranean-style pasta, fish, and meat cooked without fat.

OUTSTANDING TREATMENTS
Thermal Mud and Hydromassage.

ACTIVITIES
Horseback Riding (at nearby country club); Golf (driving range and putting green); and Tennis.

CLASSES
Aqua-Aerobics;
Tai Chi; and
Boxing Aerobics;
(all in Italian).

NEARBY ATTRACTIONS
Shopping in Saturnia; Walking the region's three ancient hilltop towns, collectively known as the "triangle of Marema." Pitigliano is known for its tufa-rock foundation, Sovana for its ancient walls, and Sorano is famous for its gorges, fortress, and castle.

GETTING THERE
A 90-minute drive from Rome airport.

ADDRESS
58050 Saturnia
Italy

T 39-0564-601061   **F** 39-0564-601266   **E** info@termedisaturnia.it   **W** www.termedisaturnia.com

THIS SPA IS FOR YOU IF after sightseeing in Rome, you want to relax, Roman-style.

THIS SPA IS NOT FOR YOU IF you're like a cat and hate soaking in water; or you absolutely cannot tolerate the smell of sulfur.

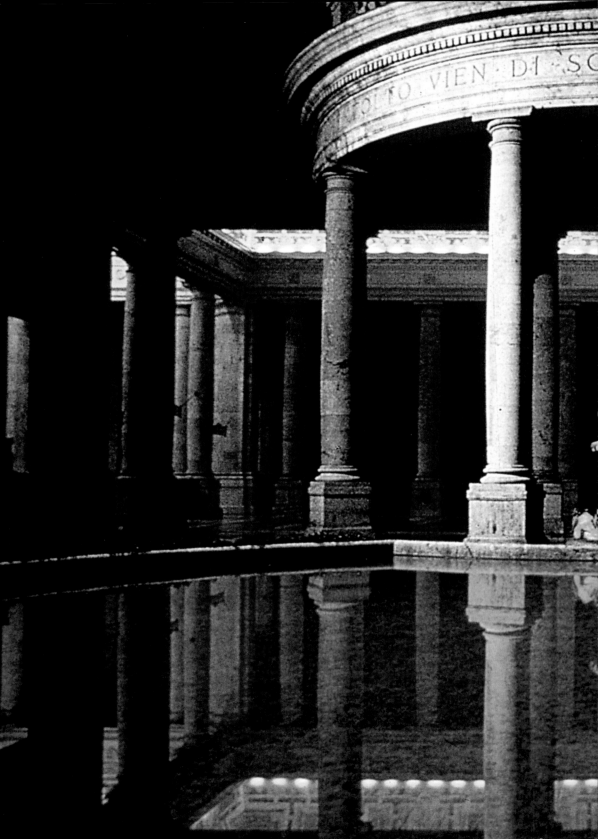

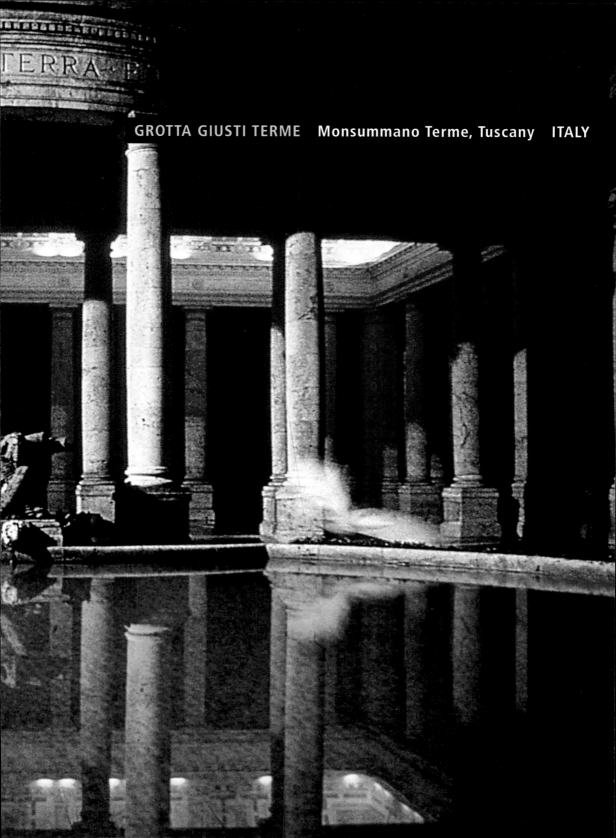

GROTTA GIUSTI TERME   Monsummano Terme, Tuscany   ITALY

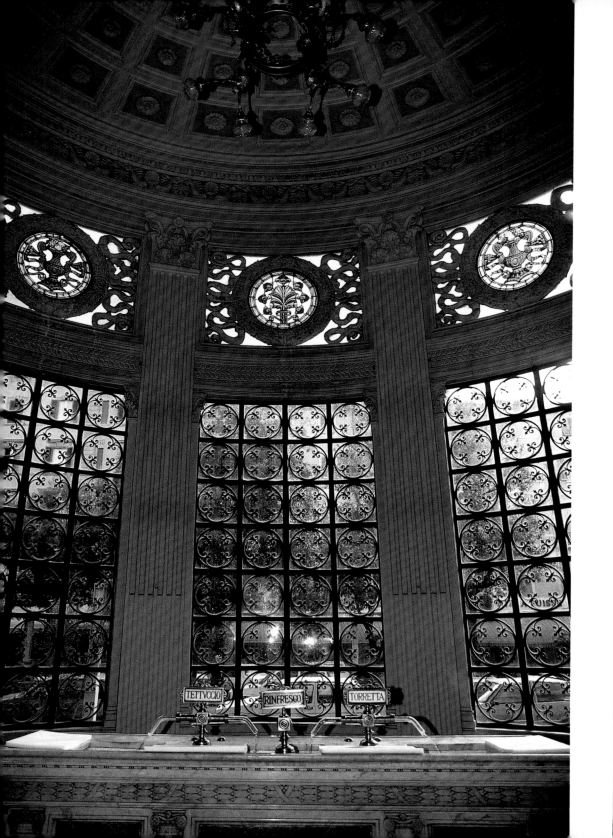

GROTTA GIUSTI TERME, MONSUMMANO TERME, TUSCANY, ITALY

On my third day at Grotta Giusti, I finally get around to ordering from the sparse spa menu. "I'll try the egg-white omelet," I tell the waiter, whose aggressive and operatic gestures remind me of my grandfather, an Italian waiter who worked at New York's Plaza Hotel for thirty years.

"No, no, no, *signora*," he tells me, shaking his head and grimacing, just as my grandfather would have done—he had very definite opinions on food.

"You don't want that. No taste. Try the fish."

"I really want to try the spa menu."

Suddenly, I have a flashback of being six years old and my grandfather plying me with food. "*Signorina bella bambina*," he would say. "Try some...Teh! Teh! Don't you know what's good?" Unfortunately, he'd be holding up a forkful of something resembling pickled sea urchins and my lips would be defiantly sealed.

As an adult I find it hard to refuse food. And I know from personal experience that there's no sense arguing with an Italian waiter on the subject. I agree to the fish.

"And I'll bring you the pasta. It's very fresh," says the waiter. "Just a small bowl, don't worry."

That's spa food, Italian-style. If you don't keep going back for seconds, it's just as healthy as the best gourmet American spa food, and you may even lose a few pounds. Nutritionists recommend a Mediterranean diet, and its liberal use of olive oil, fresh fruit, and vegetables.

My waiter was right. The sea bass was perfect, moist, and mouth-watering, and the pasta light, fluffy, and at the same time, substantial. Like most Tuscan food, everything at Grotta Giusti is simple, fresh and vibrantly flavorful, with just the right hint of garlic, a sprinkle of olive oil, and perhaps a basil leaf tossed in.

The cuisine is not the only star attraction. Nestled in the lush Tuscan foothills, this former home of nineteenth-century poet Giuseppe Giusti conceals some of the earth's most spectacular steam baths—the largest thermal grotto in the world.

Have you ever wanted to take shelter in a cave for some peace and quiet? This is the place to do it. On entering this underground paradise, you are greeted by a hostess, as if you've just arrived at a romantic restaurant that happens to be inside a volcano. Icicle-shaped stalactites hang from the roof of the cave, but lounge chairs and soft yellow lights give the place a homey feel, inviting you to relax, work up a sweat, and perhaps fantasize rugged faces in the carved rock. The sound of water, seeping from the walls and trickling to the floor, echoes throughout the cave. Guests wander by in hooded robes, looking like medieval monks. The steam carries such minerals as bicarbonate-sulfate, calcium, and magnesium—believed to be beneficial for arthritis and respiratory ailments. After only twenty minutes perspiring in this exotic underworld spa, the skin is incredibly soft. The cave extends almost a thousand feet and is divided into three parts: paradise (the coolest), purgatory, and hell (with a temperature reaching as high as 100 degrees Fahrenheit). Although the caves are primarily a place for lounging, guests can also scuba dive in an underground lake.

In lieu of a shower, guests might opt for a Scotch spray—a hosing-down performed by an attendant using water of varying degrees of force. I had my first Scotch shower after a transatlantic flight and it soothed my muscles and jolted me out of jet lag.

Grotta Giusti is only a fifteen-minute ride to Montecatini, the spa town made famous by the Romans and the Fellini film *8 1/2*. Concrete-block buildings from the seventies contrast with the rambling green spa park, a place of grand neo-Renaissance temples and hydrotherapy centers that still invite one to "take the waters." The ancient Romans believed the waters to be a cure for liver maladies,

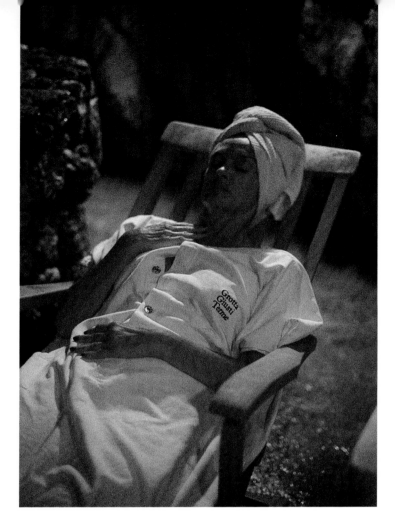

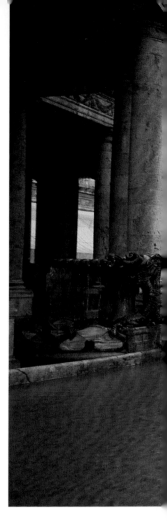

digestive disorders, and gynecological problems. Every year, some 300,000 people still visit the town, sampling the waters and taking a stroll (walking being part of the cure) through the lushly landscaped park. The Tettucio building, named after one of the springs, is the pump room, with an interior that suggests a giant marble opera house. Beneath a classical rotunda, the orchestra plays an aria as visitors fill their glasses from ornate gold faucets flowing with water from five different springs. As the waters can have a purgative effect, the Tettucio is outfitted with countless meticulously maintained bathrooms. One can also enjoy a mud treatment at some of the other spa buildings. Mud is added to the thermal waters, and machines resembling cement mixers churn it for up to six months in order to achieve the desired consistency.

After sipping the water from the Tettucio spring, I was reminded of Charles Dickens' description of the waters at Bath, which, he declared, "tasted like warm flatirons." Only an Italian waiter—or my grandfather—could persuade me to drink more.

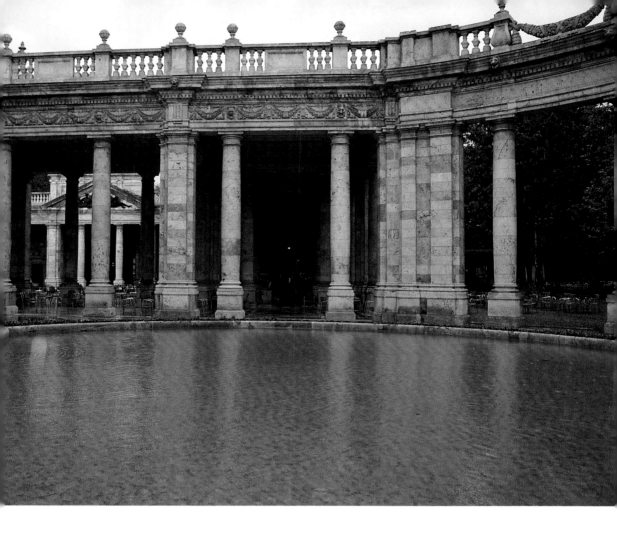

PRICE $–$$

ROOMS 70
Some basic, clean & pleasant. Others elegantly appointed.

FOOD
Outstanding, fresh and delicious Tuscan fare in main restaurant.

OUTSTANDING TREATMENTS
Fango (mud packs) and Steam Bath in the grotto.

CLASSES
Aqua-Aerobics; Tai Chi; and Yoga.

NEARBY ATTRACTIONS
Florence, Pisa, Siena, Lucca, San Gimignano, and Via Reggio beaches.

GETTING THERE
About an hour's drive or train ride from Florence.

ADDRESS
Via Grotta Giusti, 11411
51015 Monsummano Terme, Italy

T 39-0572-90771   **F** 39-0572-9077300   **E** info@grottagiustispa.com   **W** www.grottagiustispa.com

THIS SPA IS FOR YOU IF you yearn for the hills of Tuscany, a good sweat, and delicious Italian food.
THIS SPA IS NOT FOR YOU IF caves give you the creeps.

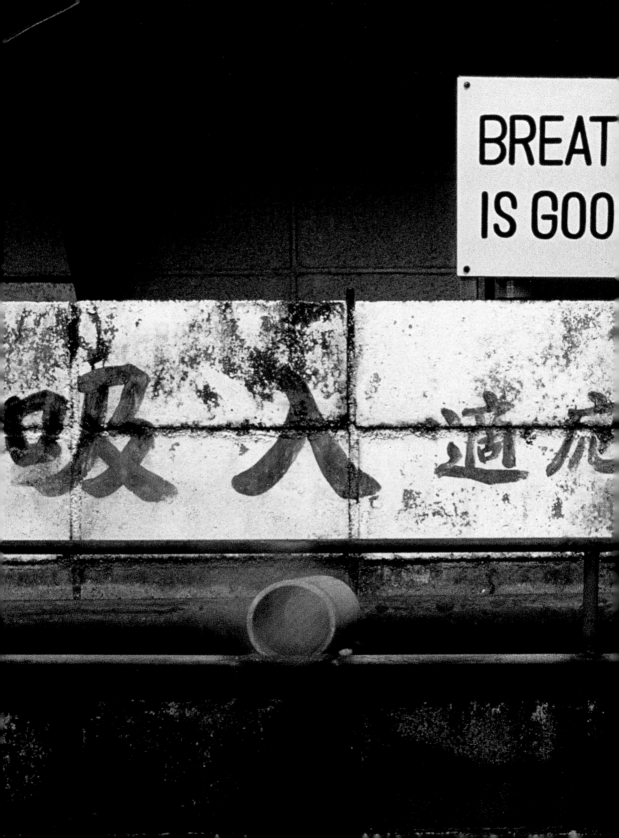

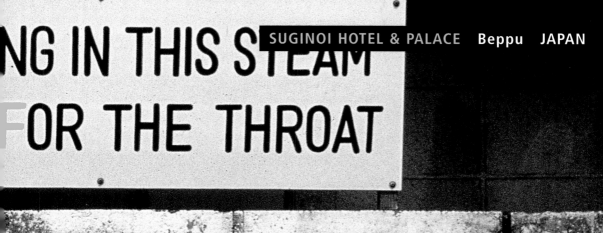

NG IN THIS STEAM

FOR THE THROAT

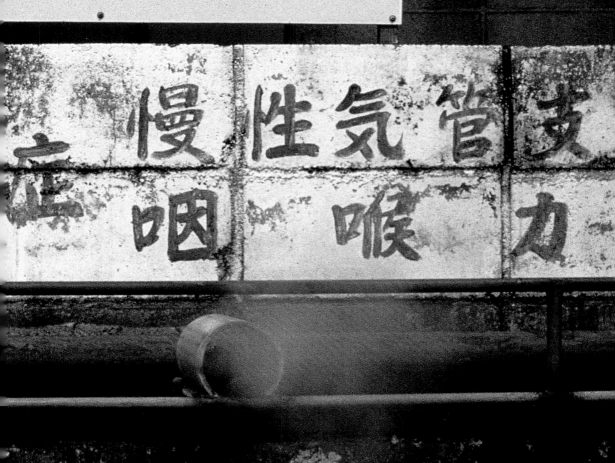

SUGINOI HOTEL & PALACE, BEPPU, JAPAN

Every kid knows the pleasure of going to the beach and burying himself in a snug cocoon of sand, and then joyfully bursting free from it. In the city of Beppu, Japan's largest hot springs spa destination on the southern island of Kyushu, burrowing in the sand is serious business for those of all ages. The Takegawara Bathhouse is world-famous for its sand treatments, where you lie supine in a hole while an attendant pours buckets of sand over you up to your neck. The sand is moistened using the region's abundant mineral waters, and creates a warm, earthen poultice to soothe muscle soreness and aching joints. Sand baths are a traditional treatment for arthritis, and circulatory and digestive problems. After fifteen minutes, you're ready for a plunge into the *onsen*, Japanese for "hot springs."

Japan sits atop a ring of fire—the same churning, subterranean heat that produced the volcanic archipelago in prehistoric times. The land is rich with onsen, some 30,000 in all, and over the centuries a highly developed culture of bathing has evolved. It is said that Americans bathe to get clean, but the Japanese get clean to bathe. Hot springs are the primary tourist destination among the Japanese, the second being theme parks.

Gaudy Beppu is a little of both. With its arcades, indoor beaches, and monkey park, it is often called "the Las Vegas of Japan." It boasts the largest volume of thermal water anywhere in the world, and when one approaches the city on a cool day, funnels of steam can be seen rising up like tantalizing ghosts. Those accustomed to U.S. and European spas be forewarned: spa life here is all about the bathing. There are no Pilates classes, no jazz aerobics, no aromatherapy wraps.

There is, however, a tour of *jigoku*—Japanese for "hell." In actuality, jigoku is composed of nine thermal water pools, or separate hells; too hot to bathe in, but incredibly beautiful to look at. The effect is reminiscent of a Salvador Dalí painting crossed with a postcard from Yellowstone National Park. A few "hells" stand out: "Blood Hell," scarlet red from melted clay; "Sea Hell," a sheen of cobalt blue; and "Tornado Hell," which features a geyser that shoots out a steady stream of scalding water every twenty-five minutes.

Though the thermal baths are a bit cooler than hell, they're more than hot enough. The Japanese have an expression for bathing in steaming hot water, *yudedako*, which translates as "boiled octopus." Some Japanese enjoy plunging into 110-degree Fahrenheit baths (screaming on impact is encouraged), and emerging lobster-red a few minutes later. It's claimed this treatment helps one attain mental clarity and, in rare cases, enlightenment.

An ancient legend about the Beppu springs tells of a Shinto deity named Sukunahiko who was cured of illness after another deity plunged him into the waters. In the ninth century, it was written that when you "take a dip, you look more attractive than ever. When you take another, you suffer from no illness for the rest of your life."

Onsen and adjoining inns, or *ryokan*, are numerous in Beppu, and are wonderful spots for cultural observations. The small neighborhood onsen are where many locals meet and chat, much like a cafe. At the other end of the scale is the most famous bathhouse in town, the Suginoi Palace (part of the Suginoi Hotel), which houses two pools in a space the size of an airplane hanger. The hotel has great views of the city, but its charm is kitschy. There are sound-and-light shows, video arcades, circuses, and a food court. It's also a great place to take the kids. Nudity is customary in the sex-segregated baths, and bashful Americans may prefer Aqua Beat, a water park with slides, a simulated wave pool, and a sand beach. There you can bury yourself in the sand, as you did when you were a kid. But it's a far cry from a sand treatment at a proper Japanese bathhouse.

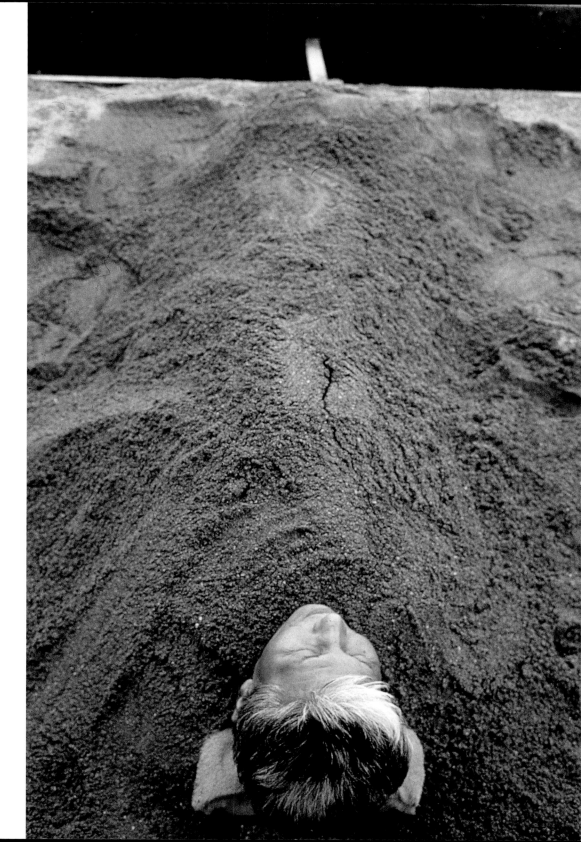

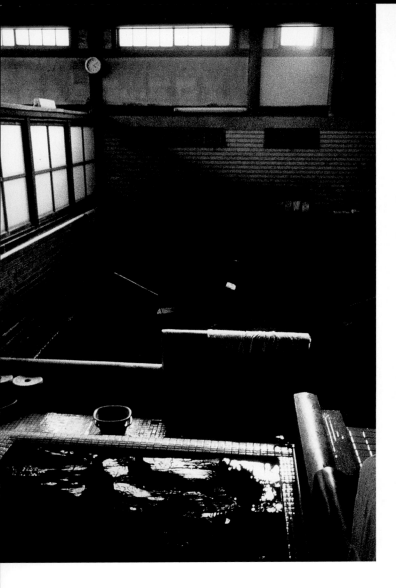

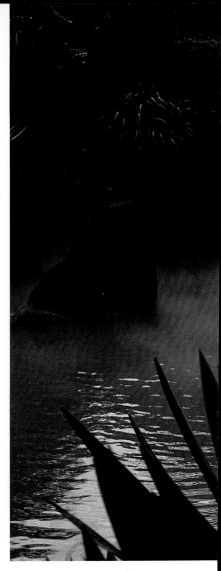

PRICE $$–$$$

ROOMS 574
Basic, clean & pleasant.
Some Western-style
and some Japanese with
tatami mats.

FOOD
Six restaurants; an
all-you-can eat buffet;

French; Japanese;
Western; gourmet seafood
restaurant; McDonald's.

**OUTSTANDING
TREATMENTS**
Sand Bath.

ACTIVITIES
Bathing is the
main attraction.

NEARBY ATTRACTIONS
The geothermal wonders
known as "the hells"
(see text); monkey park.

FOR CHILDREN
An indoor water park with
a wave pool; bowling;
video arcade.

GETTING THERE
About a 90-minute drive
from Oita airport, which is
a 40-minute flight from
Tokyo.

ADDRESS
Kankaiji 1, Beppu City,
Oita Prefecture
Japan

T 81-977-24-1161   **F** 81-977-26-7707   **E** info@suginoi-hotel.com   **W** www.suginoi-hotel.com/index_e.html

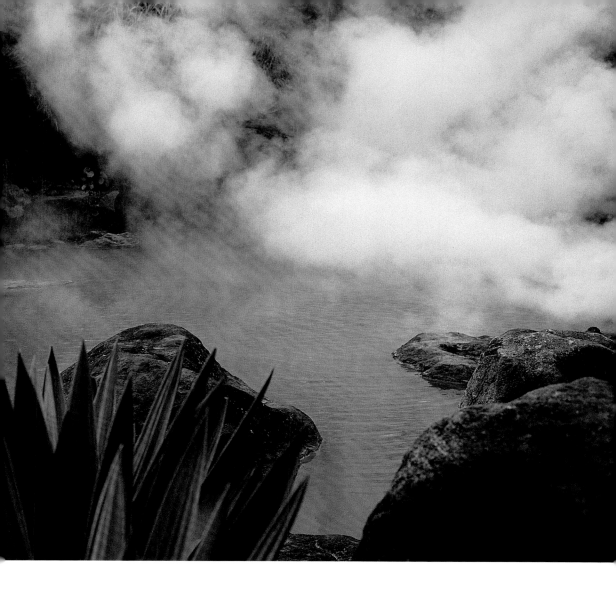

THIS SPA IS FOR YOU IF you love hot springs and are interested in Japanese bathing culture.

THIS SPA IS NOT FOR YOU IF you want a convenient spot from Tokyo.

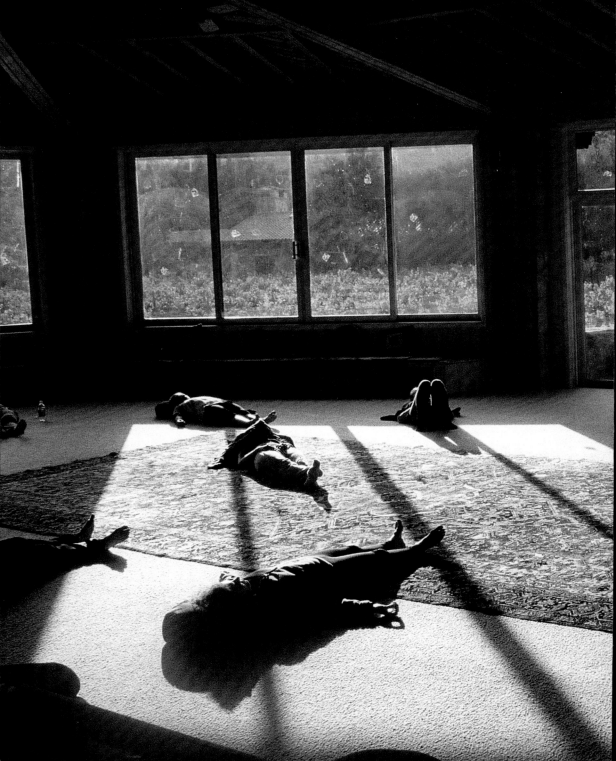

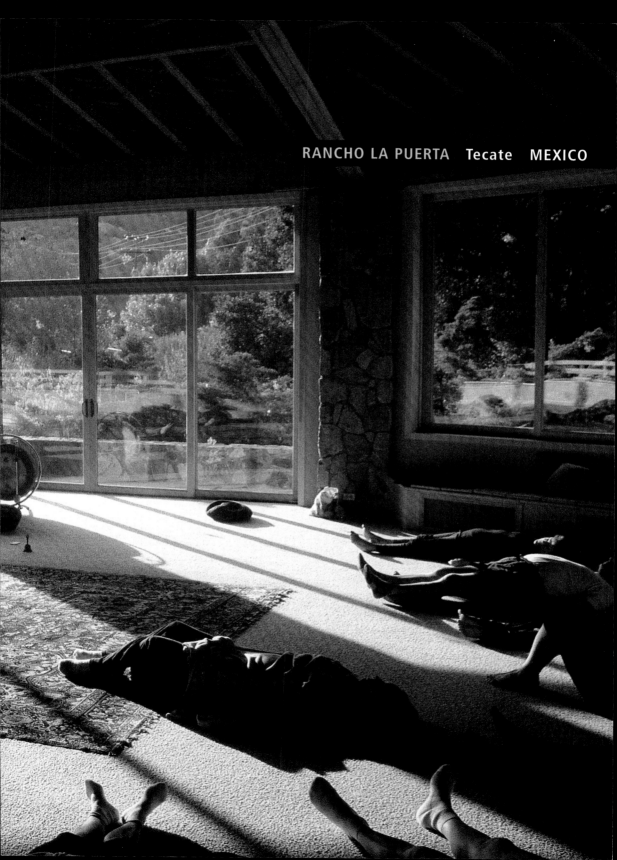

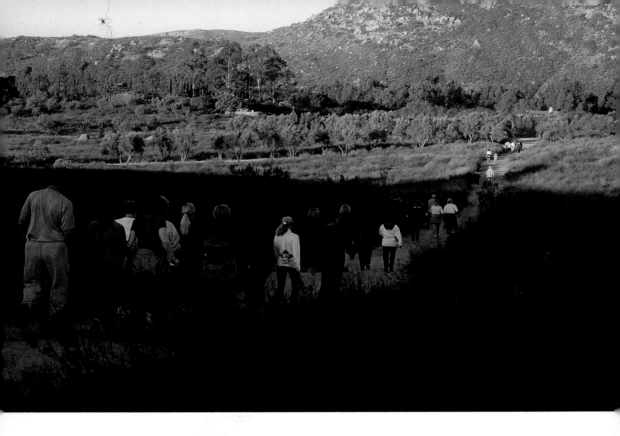

PRICE $$$–$$$$

ROOMS
Accommodates 160 guests in *rancheras* (studio bedrooms with bath), haciendas, villa studios, and suites. Some are basic, clean & pleasant, others elegantly appointed. No TV. A few rooms have phones.

FOOD
The main dining room offers a buffet breakfast and lunch. Dinners are served by waitstaff. Most entrées are vegetarian; occasionally fish and chicken are offered. Some say the fresh, low-fat cuisine— heavy on grains and legumes—leaves them hungry. Others are pleasantly sated. The heavy vegetarian fare can leave some reaching for Beano (which is served alongside the salt). No alcohol, with the exception of wine served on the last night.

OUTSTANDING TREATMENTS
Hot Stone Massage and Craniosacral Massage.

CLASSES
A huge selection of fitness classes. Yoga (all levels); African Dance; Boxing. Arts and Crafts: Herbal Wreath-Making; Jewelry-Making; and Painting.

ACTIVITIES
Hiking; Walking the Labyrinth (see The Golden Door, page 24); and Tennis. Evening lectures and workshops vary from week to week. A sample selection: The Power of Rituals in Daily Life; Discovering the Writer in You; Everything You always Wanted to Know about Hypnosis.

GETTING THERE
About an hour's drive from San Diego. On Saturdays, a chartered bus picks up guests at the airport free of charge.

ADDRESS
Tecate, Baja California, Mexico

MAILING ADDRESS
PO Box 463057
Escondido, CA
92046-3057

T 800-443-7565   **F** 760-744-4222   **E** reservations@rancholapuerta.com   **W** www.rancholapuerta.com

THIS SPA IS FOR YOU IF you love meditation, fitness, meeting new people, and vegetarian food.
THIS SPA IS NOT FOR YOU IF you're into pure pampering, sightseeing, and margaritas.

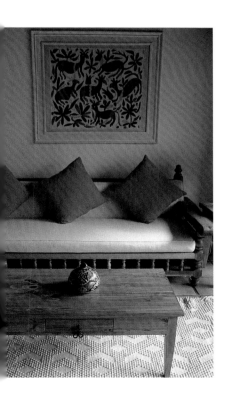

RANCHO LA PUERTA, TECATE, MEXICO

Rancho La Puerta is a little slice of self-improvement paradise. Yes, this Mexican desert enclave has palm trees and crystal-clear swimming pools, and a majestic purple mountain that looms protectively nearby, but that's only part of what makes it paradise for the hundreds of guests who return year after year. This is the quintessential training ground for both body and soul; it's not surprising that there have been as many as eight Oprah sightings over the years.

All guests must arrive on a Saturday, and they might be overwhelmed at first by the array of classes and activities. Planning the required seven-day stay is a bit like being a college freshman, dropping and adding courses. All levels of yoga are offered—in fact, Rancho La Puerta attracts some of the best teachers in the United States—along with African dancing, Pilates, and a host of creative activities. You may say to yourself: "I've always wanted to try that." Whether it be herbal wreath-making, jewelry-making, or a meditation dinner, a stay here offers just the opportunity to do things you thought you never had time for.

Or even things you never considered. One type-A editor in his mid-forties confided to me that he enjoyed the herbal wreath-making class. "It wasn't so much about making the wreath, it was the whole experience," he said. "Music was playing in the background and the smell of the herbs was really pleasant. It was more about unwinding and slowing down, a meditative experience."

Opportunities for meditative experiences abound, especially during a morning hike at the base of Mount Kuchumaa, a place considered sacred by the local Indians. Some of the nightly lectures and workshops, like the one I attended on the importance of rituals, offer meditative time as well. I met one young woman who was in a great deal of pain over the murder of her mother; she had broken down crying as others in the workshop tried to comfort her. The next morning I spotted her sitting on a rock facing Mount Kuchumaa, breathing deeply, looking very much at peace.

Rancho's owner, Deborah Szekely, credits the mountain with special mystical powers, and attributes the spa's success over the years to them. "It keeps drawing visitors back," she says. Deborah and her husband Edmond came to this desert spot in 1940 with the goal of setting up a "health camp," making Rancho the first modern-day spa in North America. Edmond would give lectures on spirituality, philosophy, and nutrition, and in between guests would hike, do calisthenics, take dance classes, and partake of simple low-calorie meals from the organic garden. One activity was tending the crops.

Today, dinner at Rancho can be a solitary or social affair—it's your choice to be seated at a large table or not. I met several groups of women who use the spa as a site for annual reunions. (Many return with their husbands.) "It's such a special place for us," says one. "We unwind and support one another, for whatever is happening in our lives."

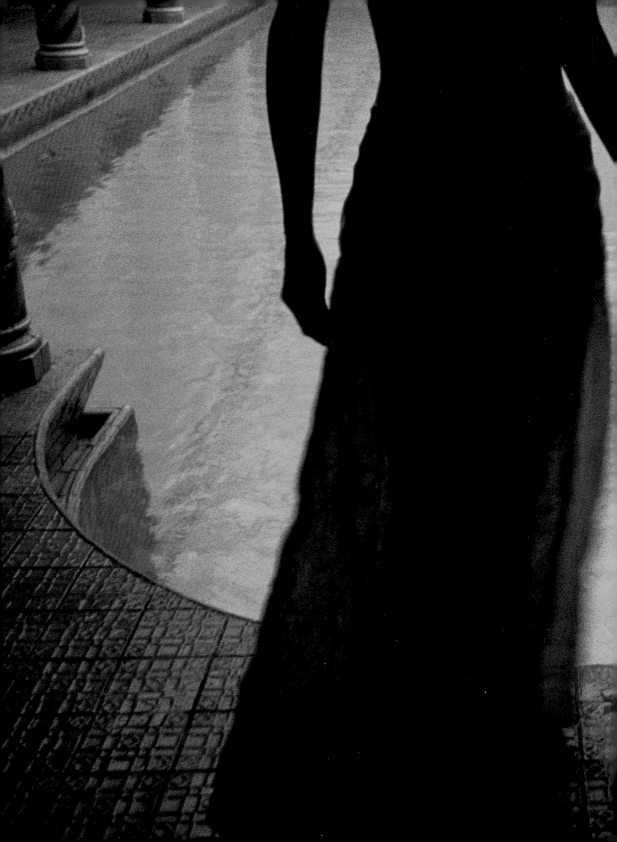

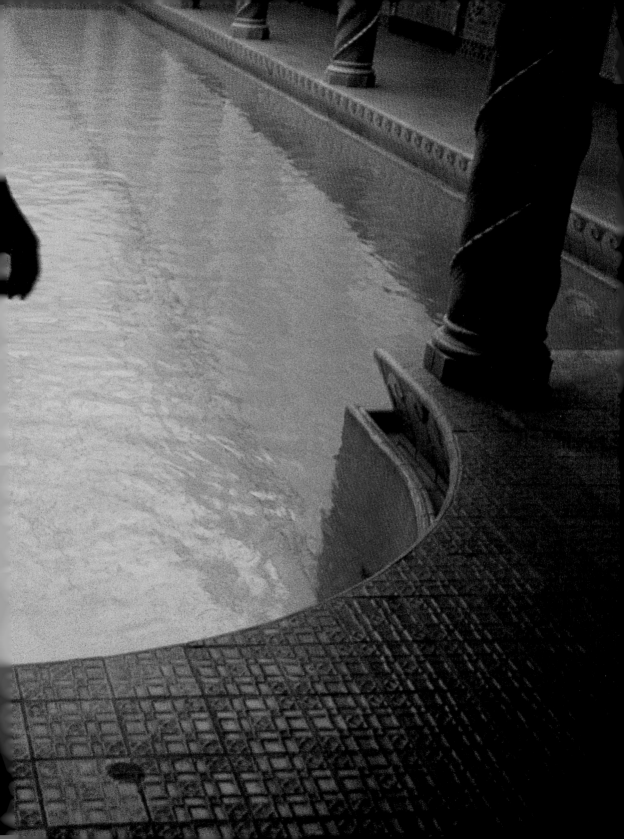

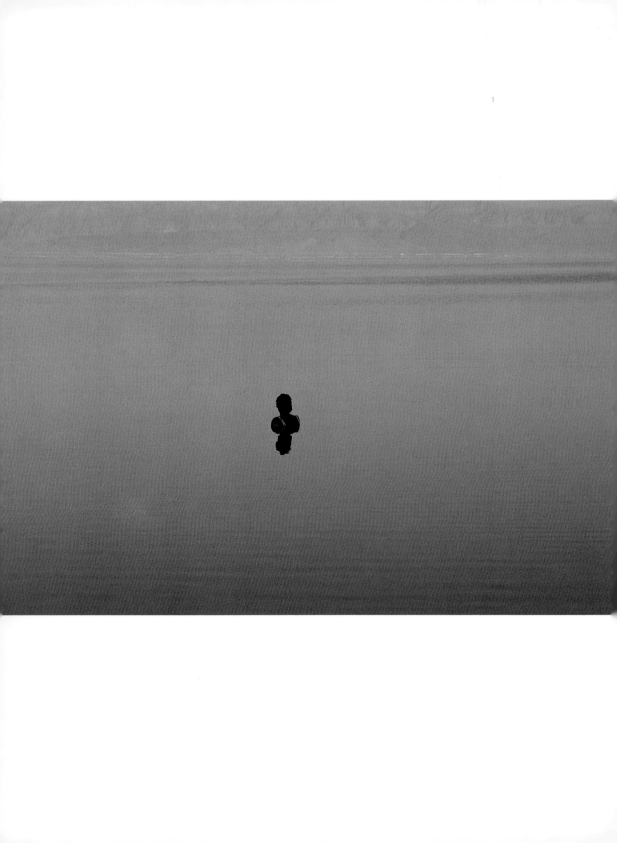

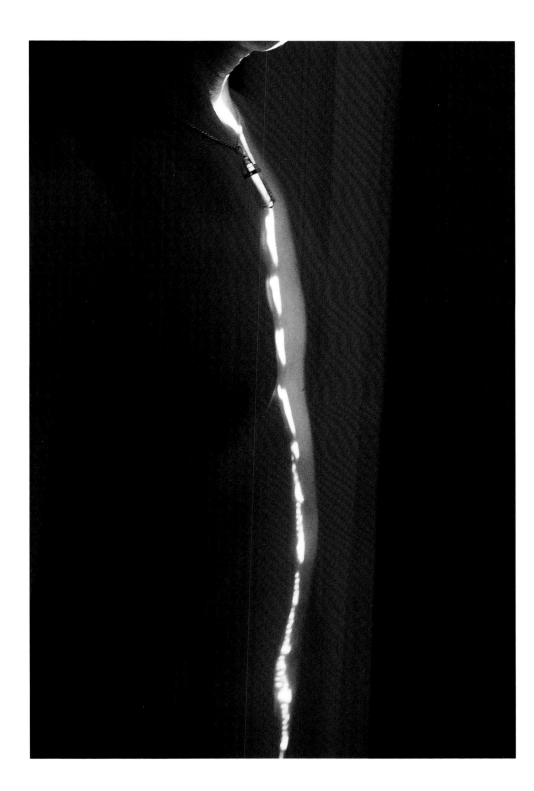

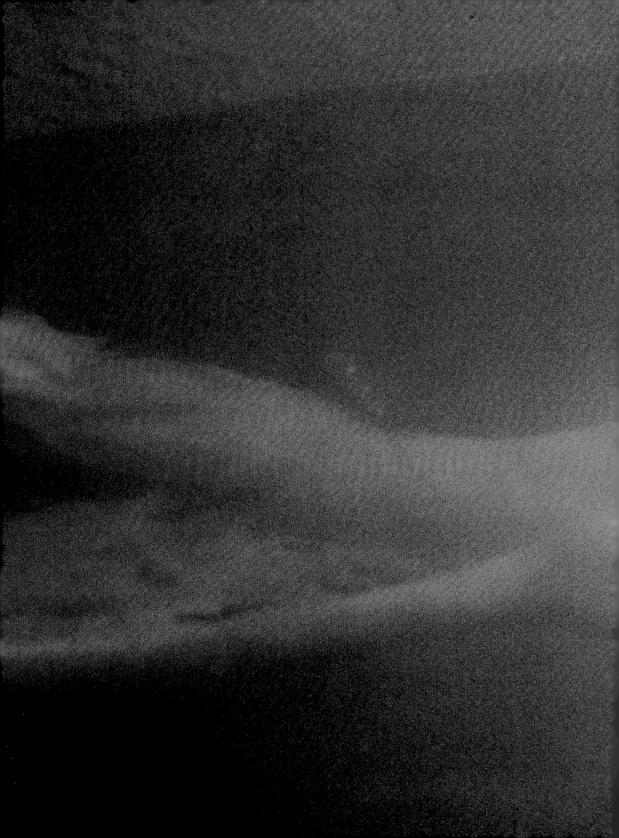

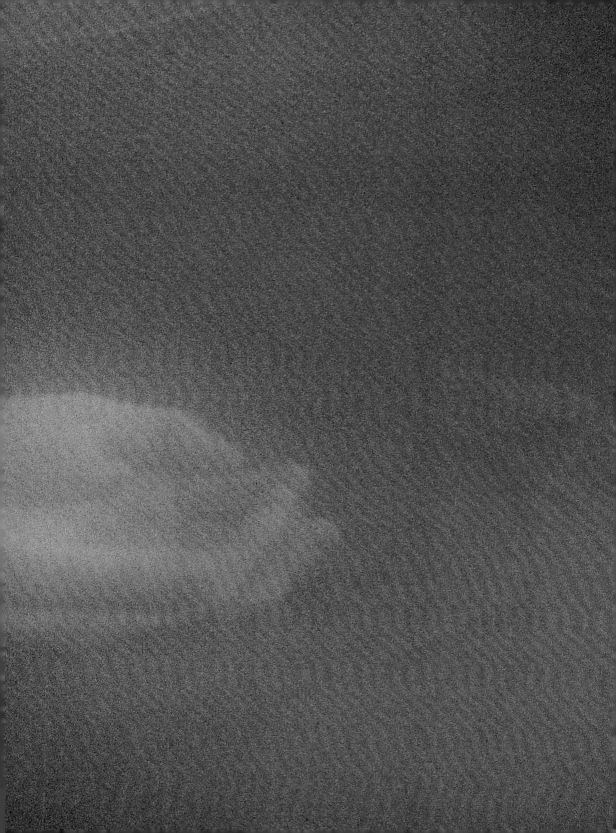

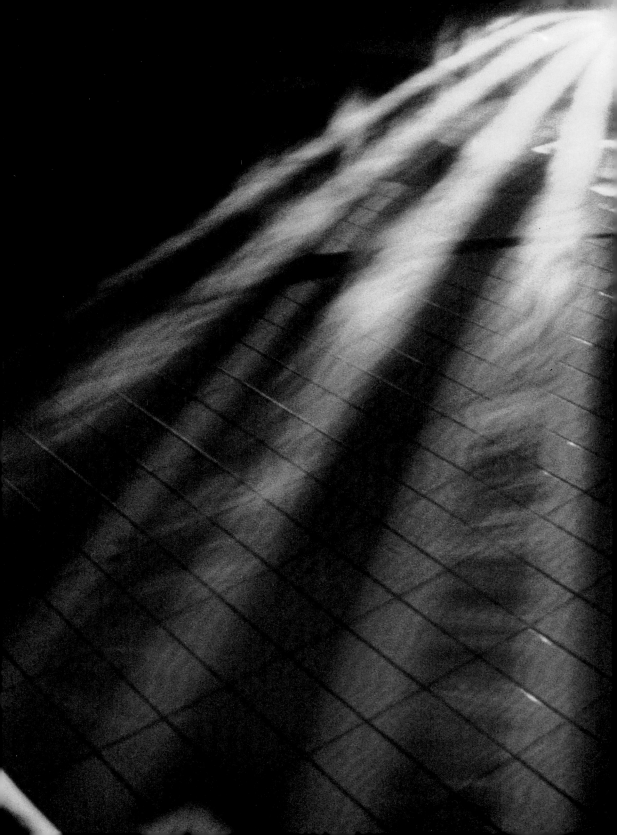

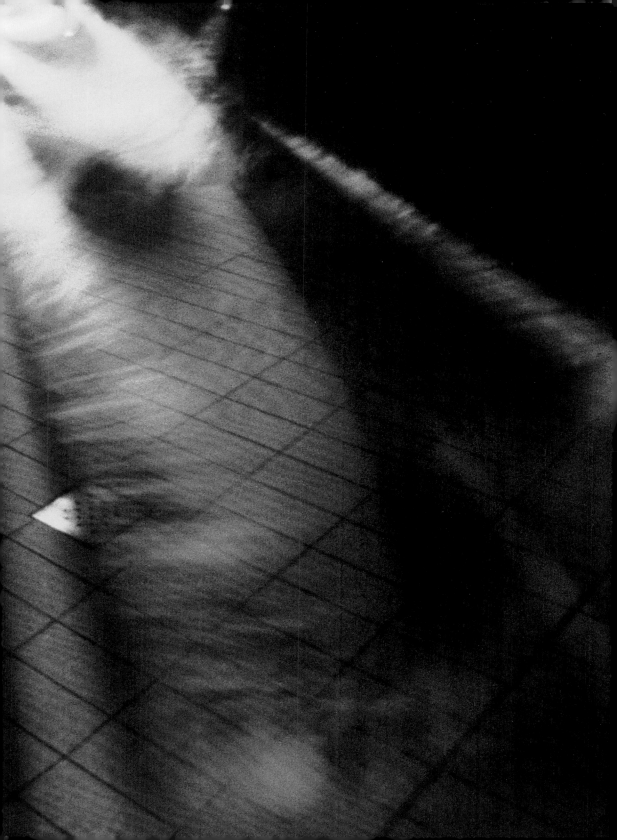

Captions

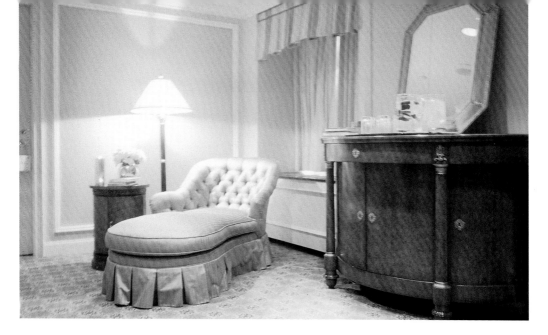

We would like to thank everyone in the spa and healing business who helped in the preparation of this book, as well as all the spa-goers who shared their personal experiences with us. Special thanks to Marion Schneider, Klaus Boehm, and Micky Remann of Toskana Therme; Dr. Milada Sarova of Karlovy Vary; Brian and Anna Maria Clement of Hippocrates Health Institute; Mary Elizabeth Gifford and Sue Annetts of the Rancho La Puerta and the Golden Door; Kurotel's Luciana Bahia for being such a gracious host; Pat Eli of Hilton Waikoloa Village for her Aloha spirit; and Miraval's cowboy shrink Wyatt Webb and Dr. Tim Frank for their innovative approaches to healing. Thanks also to *Spa Finder*'s Malcolm Abrams for bringing us together.

Linda would like to thank Anne Tucker of the Museum of Fine Arts, Houston, and Dr. Barbara Wally of the Summer Art Academy, Salzburg. Bernie Burt, of the International Spa Association, and Pamela Price were generous enough to present exhibitions of her work at ISPA Europe and at the Spa Soirée at Spa Esmerelda in Palm Springs, California. A big thank-you to Lothar Voeller for his loving support and his talented photo assistance.

Annette would like to thank Malcolm Abrams, Frank van Putten, and all the folks at *Spa Finder* for introducing her to spas as something more than just pampering retreats; Kate Klise for her vicarious spa enthusiasm and editorial eagle eye; Bill Corsa at Specialty Book Marketing for his wise counsel; Anne Hardy for her priceless friendship and good advice. And to her husband, Chuck, for his loving encouragement and brilliance. She hopes someday he will try a Pilates class.

Linda and Annette also wish to thank powerHouse's Susanne König for her support and editorial vision for the book, and Yuko Uchikawa for a brilliant design and unfailing professionalism.

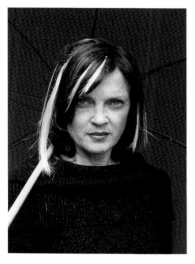

Lothar Voeller

Linda Troeller is a fine art and editorial photographer whose books include *The Erotic Lives of Women* (Scalo, 1998) (which was called "gutsy and imaginative" by *The New York Times*) and *Healing Waters* (Aperture, 1998), which won the Book Award for Excellence in 1999 from Pictures of the Year. She also won first place for Magazine/Pictorial from Pictures of the Year in 1992 for a photograph that later appeared in *Healing Waters*. Her photo-collage exhibition of "TB-AIDS Diary" won the Ferguson Award in 1989. She lives in New York City, and teaches workshops and has exhibitions worldwide. She has created a Spa Picture Archive, which provides photos for decor, brochures, and magazine articles on spa treatments and healing. For more information on her archive, contact www.lindatroeller.com.

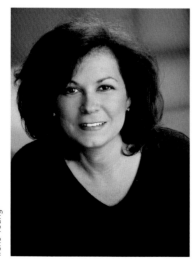

Irene Young

Annette Foglino is an award-winning journalist who has reported on everything from women's health to youth violence, the Mafia, and rehabilitation of prostitutes. Her features on these and other subjects have appeared in *New York* Magazine, *Reader's Digest*, *Glamour*, and many other national publications. A former reporter for *Life* magazine, she has also written lifestyle and travel articles for *Self*, *Marie Claire*, *Shape*, and *Living Fit*. As a contributing editor to *Spa Finder* magazine, she has written extensively on the mind-body connection and spa travel. She lives in New York City, but continues to cover travel destinations and social issues all over the world.

SPA JOURNEYS

Published in the United States by powerHouse Books,
a division of powerHouse Cultural Entertainment, Inc.
68 Charlton Street, New York, NY 10014-4601
telephone 212 604 9074, fax 212 366 5247
e-mail: spajourneys@powerHouseBooks.com
web site: www.powerHouseBooks.com

First edition, 2004

Library of Congress Cataloging-in-Publication Data:

Troeller, Linda
    Spa journeys / photographs by Linda Troeller ; text by Annette Foglino.-- 1st ed.
    p. cm.
    ISBN 1-57687-190-8
    1. Health resorts. I. Foglino, Annette, 1960- II. Title.

RA794.T76 2003
613'.122--dc21

2003051725

Hardcover ISBN 1-57687-190-8

Separations, printing, and binding by Sfera International, Milan

A complete catalog of powerHouse Books and
Limited Editions is available upon request;
please call, write, or be rejuvenated on our web site.

10 9 8 7 6 5 4 3 2 1

Printed and bound in Italy

Book design by Yuko Uchikawa